Judith L. Howe, PhD
Editor

Older People and Their Caregivers Across the Spectrum of Care

Older People and Their Caregivers Across the Spectrum of Care has been co-published simultaneously as *Journal of Gerontological Social Work*, Volume 40, Numbers 1/2 2002.

Pre-publication REVIEWS, COMMENTARIES, EVALUATIONS . . .

"**C**OMPREHENSIVE. . . . A VAL- UABLE TEACHING RESOURCE for educators in a wide range of fields. . . . Dr. Howe has compiled an excellent collection of chapters spanning the evolution of geriatric assessment and caregiving issues."

Andrea Sherman, PhD
Project Director
The Consortium of New York
Geriatric Education Centers
Division of Nursing
The Steinhardt School of Education
New York University

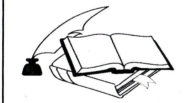

More Pre-publication
REVIEWS, COMMENTARIES, EVALUATIONS . . .

"THIS FINE BOOK will serve well as A TEXTBOOK FOR TRAINING PROFESSIONAL CARE-GIVERS as well as A FIELD MANUAL FOR THOSE PROVIDING THE CARE. Readers will discover what social caseworkers have long known: older persons do not need special care merely because they are older, but because they are vulnerable to a complex variety of social factors, physical problems, emotional needs, and loss of personal autonomy. Judith Howe and the contributors to this book are to be commended for making available a compendium of resources that brings together in one volume THE LATEST RESEARCH AND MODELS OF CARE FOR AN AGING POPULATION."

Ray S. Anderson, PhD
*Senior Professor
of Theology and Ministry
Fuller Theological Seminary*

"IMPORTANT. . . . Offers critical information in several important areas of practice with older adults and their caregivers. Beginning with a superb chapter by Dr. Barbara Berkman and her colleagues on the need to revisit our ideas of assessment of older adults, the book includes chapters that address programs for older persons who are abused as well as several interesting chapters on programs for caregivers. It is my belief that this book will become a staple for those practicing gerontological social work because it offers information that WILL ASSIST PRACTITIONERS IN IDENTIFYING BEST PRACTICES. Furthermore, the book offers the information necessary to implement these programs. . . . A VITAL STEP in establishing the social work role in working with older adults."

Gregory J. Paveza, PhD, MSW
*Professor
School of Social Work
and President
Faculty Senate
University of South Florida, Tampa*

The Haworth Social Work Practice Press
An Imprint of The Haworth Press, Inc.

Older People and Their Caregivers Across the Spectrum of Care

Older People and Their Caregivers Across the Spectrum of Care has been co-published simultaneously as *Journal of Gerontological Social Work*, Volume 40, Numbers 1/2 2002.

The *Journal of Gerontological Social Work* Monographic "Separates"

Below is a list of "separates," which in serials librarianship means a special issue simultaneously published as a special journal issue or double-issue *and* as a "separate" hardbound monograph. (This is a format which we also call a "DocuSerial.")

"Separates" are published because specialized libraries or professionals may wish to purchase a specific thematic issue by itself in a format which can be separately cataloged and shelved, as opposed to purchasing the journal on an on-going basis. Faculty members may also more easily consider a "separate" for classroom adoption.

"Separates" are carefully classified separately with the major book jobbers so that the journal tie-in can be noted on new book order slips to avoid duplicate purchasing.

You may wish to visit Haworth's Website at . . .

http://www.HaworthPress.com

. . . to search our online catalog for complete tables of contents of these separates and related publications. You may also call 1-800-HAWORTH (outside US/Canada: 607-722-5857), or Fax 1-800-895-0582 (outside US/Canada: 607-771-0012), or e-mail at:

docdelivery@haworthpress.com

Older People and Their Caregivers Across the Spectrum of Care, edited by Judith L. Howe, PhD (Vol. 40, No. 1/2, 2002). *Focuses on numerous issues relating to caregiving and social work assessment for improving quality of life for the elderly.*

Advancing Gerontological Social Work Education, edited by M. Joanna Mellor, DSW and Joann Ivry, PhD (Vol. 39, No. 1/2, 2002). *Examines the current status of geriatric/gerontological education; offers models for curriculum development within the classroom and the practice arena.*

erontological Social Work Practice: Issues, Challenges, and Potential, edited by Enid Opal Cox, DSW, Elizabeth S. Kelchner, MSW, ACSW, and Rosemary Chapin, PhD, MSW (Vol. 36, No. 3/4, 2001). *This book gives you an essential overview of the role, status, and potential of ?erontological social work in aging societies around the world. Drawing on the expertise of 'aders in the field, it identifies key policy and practice issues and suggests directions for the fu- ·e. Here you'll find important perspectives on home health care, mental health, elder abuse, 'er workers' issues, and death and dying, as well as an examination of the policy and practice 's of utmost concern to social workers dealing with the elderly.*

'ork Practice with the Asian American Elderly, edited by Namkee G. Choi, PhD (Vol. ., 1/2, 2001). *"Encompasses the richness of diversity among Asian Americans by including on Vietnamese, Japanese, Chinese, Taiwanese, Asian Indian, and Korean Americans."* R. Hooyman, PhD, MSW, Professor and Dean Emeritus, University of Washington 'Social Work, Seattle)

as Carers of Children with Disabilities: Facing the Challenges, edited by Philip PhD, ACSW, and Matthew Janicki, PhD (Vol. 33, No. 3, 2000). *Here is the first ve consideration of the unique needs and experiences of grandparents caring for developmental disabilities. The vital information found here will assist administrators, and policymakers to include the needs of this special population g and delivery of services, and it will help grandparents in this situation to better elves as well as for the children in their charge.*

d the Twenty-First Century: Issues and Challenges for Culturally Competent Practice, edited by Melvin Delgado, PhD (Vol. 30, No. 1/2, 1998). *Explores the l gerontological social work will encounter as it attempts to meet the needs of the er of Latino elders utilizing culturally competent principles.*

ge, edited by Rose Dobrof, DSW, and Harry R. Moody, PhD (Vol. 29, No. 2/3, nges us to uphold the right to age with dignity, which is embedded in the heart* *and soul of every man and woman." (H. James Towey, President, Commission on Aging with Dignity, Tallahassee, FL)*

Intergenerational Approaches in Aging: Implications for Education, Policy and Practice, edited by Kevin Brabazon, MPA, and Robert Disch, MA (Vol. 28, No. 1/2/3, 1997). *"Provides a wealth of concrete examples of areas in which intergenerational perspectives and knowledge are needed." (Robert C. Atchley, PhD, Director, Scribbs Gerontology Center, Miami University)*

Social Work Response to the White House Conference on Aging: From Issues to Actions, edited by Constance Corley Saltz, PhD, LCSW (Vol. 27, No. 3, 1997). *"Provides a framework for the discussion of issues relevant to social work values and practice, including productive aging, quality of life, the psychological needs of older persons, and family issues." (Jordan I. Kosberg, PhD, Professor and PhD Program Coordinator, School of Social Work, Florida International University, North Miami, FL)*

Special Aging Populations and Systems Linkages, edited by M. Joanna Mellor, DSW (Vol. 25, No. 1/2, 1996). *"An invaluable tool for anyone working with older persons with special needs." (Irene Gutheil, DSW, Associate Professor, Graduate School of Social Service, Fordham University)*

New Developments in Home Care Services for the Elderly: Innovations in Policy, Program, and Practice, edited by Lenard W. Kaye, DSW (Vol. 24, No. 3/4, 1995). *"An excellent compilation. . . . Especially pertinent to the functions of administrators, supervisors, and case managers in home care. . . . Highly recommended for every home care agency and a must for administrators and middle managers." (Geriatric Nursing Book Review)*

Geriatric Social Work Education, edited by M. Joanna Mellor, DSW, and Renee Solomon, DSW (Vol. 18, No. 3/4, 1992). *"Serves as a foundation upon which educators and fieldwork instructors can build courses that incorporate more aging content." (SciTech Book News)*

Vision and Aging: Issues in Social Work Practice, edited by Nancy D. Weber, MSW (Vol. 17, No. 3/4, 1992). *"For those involved in vision rehabilitation programs, the book provides practical information and should stimulate readers to revise their present programs of care." (Journal of Vision Rehabilitation)*

Health Care of the Aged: Needs, Policies, and Services, edited by Abraham Monk, PhD (Vol. 15, No. 3/4, 1990). *"The chapters reflect firsthand experience and are competent and informative. Readers . . . will find the book rewarding and useful. The text is timely, appropriate, and well-presented." (Health & Social Work)*

Twenty-Five Years of the Life Review: Theoretical and Practical Considerations, edited by Robert Disch, MA (Vol. 12, No. 3/4, 1989). *This practical and thought-provoking book examines the history and concept of the life review.*

Gerontological Social Work: International Perspectives, edited by Merl C. Hokenstad, Jr., PhD and Katherine A. Kendall, PhD (Vol. 12, No. 1/2, 1988). *"Makes a very useful contribution in examining the changing role of the social work profession in serving the elderly." (Journal of the International Federation on Ageing)*

Gerontological Social Work Practice with Families: A Guide to Practice Issues and Service Delivery, edited by Rose Dobrof, DSW (Vol. 10, No. 1/2, 1987). *An in-depth examination of the importance of family relationships within the context of social work practice with the elderly.*

Ethnicity and Gerontological Social Work, edited by Rose Dobrof, DSW (Vol. 9, No. 4, 1987). *"Addresses the issues of ethnicity with great sensitivity. Most of the topics addressed here are rarely addressed in other literature." (Dr. Milada Disman, Department of Behavioral Science, University of Toronto)*

Social Work and Alzheimer's Disease, edited by Rose Dobrof, DSW (Vol. 9, No. 2, 1986). *"New and innovative social work roles with Alzheimer's victims and their families in both hospital and non-hospital settings." (Continuing Education Update)*

Gerontological Social Work Practice in the Community, edited by George S. Getzel, DSW and M. Joanna Mellor, DSW (Vol. 8, No. 3/4, 1985). *"A wealth of information for all practitioners who deal with the elderly. An excellent reference for faculty, administrators, clinicians, and graduate students in nursing and other service professions who work with the elderly."* *(American Journal of Care for the Aging)*

Gerontological Social Work in Home Health Care, edited by Rose Dobrof, DSW (Vol. 7, No. 4, 1984). *"A useful window onto the home health care scene in terms of current forms of service provided to the elderly and the direction of social work practice in this field today."* *(PRIDE Institute Journal)*

The Uses of Reminiscence: New Ways of Working with Older Adults, edited by Marc Kaminsky (Vol. 7, No. 1/2, 1984). *"Rich in ideas for anyone working with life review groups."* *(Guidepost)*

A Healthy Old Age: A Sourcebook for Health Promotion with Older Adults, edited by Stephanie FallCreek, MSW, and Molly K. Mettler, MSW (Vol. 6, No. 2/3, 1984). *"An outstanding text on the 'how-tos' of health promotion for elderly persons."* *(Physical Therapy)*

Gerontological Social Work Practice in Long-Term Care, edited by George S. Getzel, DSW, and M. Joanna Mellor, DSW (Vol. 5, No. 1/2, 1983). *"Veteran practitioners and graduate social work students will find the book insightful and a valuable prescriptive guide to the do's and don'ts of practice in their daily work."* *(The Gerontologist)*

Older People and Their Caregivers Across the Spectrum of Care

Judith L. Howe, PhD
Editor

Older People and Their Caregivers Across the Spectrum of Care has been co-published simultaneously as *Journal of Gerontological Social Work*, Volume 40, Numbers 1/2 2002.

The Haworth Social Work Practice Press
An Imprint of The Haworth Press, Inc.

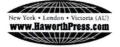

New York • London • Victoria (AU)
www.HaworthPress.com

HV
1451
.Q445
2003

Published by

The Haworth Social Work Practice Press, 10 Alice Street, Binghamton, NY 13904-1580 USA

The Haworth Social Work Practice Press is an imprint of The Haworth Press, Inc., 10 Alice Street, Binghamton, NY 13904-1580 USA.

Older People and Their Caregivers Across the Spectrum of Care has been co-published simultaneously as *Journal of Gerontological Social Work,* Volume 40, Numbers 1/2 2002.

Cover design by Jennifer Gaska.

Library of Congress Cataloging-in-Publication Data

Older people and their caregivers across the spectrum of care / Judith L. Howe.
    p. cm.
"Co-published simultaneously as Journal of gerontological social work, volume 40, numbers 1/2, 2002."
ISBN 0-7890-2283-4 (alk. paper)–ISBN 0-7890-2284-2 (soft cover: alk. paper)
    1. Aged–Care. 2. Caregivers. 3. Social work with the aged. 4. Gerontology. I. Howe, Judith L. II. Journal of gerontological social work.
HV451.0445 2004
362.6–dc22   2003015605

Indexing, Abstracting & Website/Internet Coverage

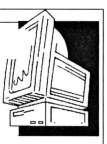

This section provides you with a list of major indexing & abstracting services. That is to say, each service began covering this periodical during the year noted in the right column. Most Websites which are listed below have indicated that they will either post, disseminate, compile, archive, cite or alert their own Website users with research-based content from this work. (This list is as current as the copyright date of this publication.)

(continued)

(continued)

* **Exact start date to come.**

continued

Special Bibliographic Notes related to special journal issues
(separates) and indexing/abstracting:

- indexing/abstracting services in this list will also cover material in any "separate" that is co-published simultaneously with Haworth's special thematic journal issue or DocuSerial. Indexing/abstracting usually covers material at the article/chapter level.
- monographic co-editions are intended for either non-subscribers or libraries which intend to purchase a second copy for their circulating collections.
- monographic co-editions are reported to all jobbers/wholesalers/approval plans. The source journal is listed as the "series" to assist the prevention of duplicate purchasing in the same manner utilized for books-in-series.
- to facilitate user/access services all indexing/abstracting services are encouraged to utilize the co-indexing entry note indicated at the bottom of the first page of each article/chapter/contribution.
- this is intended to assist a library user of any reference tool (whether print, electronic, online, or CD-ROM) to locate the monographic version if the library has purchased this version but not a subscription to the source journal.
- individual articles/chapters in any Haworth publication are also available through the Haworth Document Delivery Service (HDDS).

Older People and Their Caregivers Across the Spectrum of Care

CONTENTS

ABOUT THE EDITOR

Judith L. Howe, PhD, is Associate Professor in the Brookdale Department of Geriatrics and Adult Development at the Mount Sinai School of Medicine. She is also Associate Director for Education and Evaluation for the Bronx VA Geriatrics Research, Education and Clinic Center (GRECC) Program and Co-Director of the New York Consortium of Geriatric Education Centers. She has co-authored numerous peer-reviewed articles and book chapters on interdisciplinary education, interdisciplinary team development, and cross-disciplinary education. She is also an editor of *Ethical Patient Care: A Casebook for Geriatric Health Care Teams*, published by the Johns Hopkins University.

Dr. Howe has extensive experience in geriatric interdisciplinary education, curriculum development, aging and public policy, and administration through her work at Mount Sinai School of Medicine, the GRECC, the United States Senate, and the National Institute on Aging of the National Institutes of Health. She was Secretariat to the 1982 United Nations World Assembly on Aging. She is also a founder and chair of the board of Linkage House, a project funded by the United States Department of Housing and Urban Development for lower-income older people in East Harlem, New York. In 1980, she received the NIH Award of Merit for her work in aging. She is also a recipient of a St. Lawrence University Alumni Citation and a Fellow of the New York Academy of Medicine. Dr. Howe and her colleagues have led many workshops for health professionals geared to strengthening interdisciplinary teams and techniques for teaching teamwork. She is a member of the Gerontological Society of America, American Society on Aging, and National Association of Social Workers.

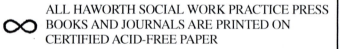

Preface

We are particularly proud to present to *Journal* readers this volume, titled *Older People and Their Caregivers Across the Spectrum of Care*, edited by Judith L. Howe, PhD, Associate Professor in the Brookdale Department of Geriatrics and Adult Development. As has been true of other volumes, this one is a marvelous reflection of the heterogeneity of the areas of expertise, experience, and interests of gerontological social workers. For many caregivers, the role is a mix of burden and fulfillment–burden, because the caregivers have other familial, work, and community responsibilities; fulfillment, because they are gratified to be able to provide care and take responsibility for functionally dependent older people, parents, siblings, spouses in their families. As the reader will see from a reading of this volume, for many caregivers, the role permits them to articulate in action their love for the care receiver. For others, the role articulates their sense of responsibility, more than their love. And as is true of many of the roles we play, there may be a mix of burden and fulfillment.

Many of the papers in this collection reflect that mix of feelings. There is, in addition, emphasis on the importance of the intricacies and requirements of the kind of assessment processes and procedures that effective service delivery to older people and their caregivers demand. Inter-professional collaboration, long-distance caregiving, and the special problem of elder abuse are among the other topics of the papers in this volume.

And finally are two reports from "The World of Practice," one on a "Friendly Companion Program," and the other about the "Stories Told and Lessons Learned" in an "Empowerment" group for Black female caregivers. We commend both of these to our readers, as wonderful examples of programs that bring meaning to the lives of the older participants.

Congratulations are due to Dr. Howe and the authors of the papers in this volume.

Rose Dobrof, Co-Editor

[Haworth co-indexing entry note]: "Preface." Dobrof, Rose. Co-published simultaneously in *Journal of Gerontological Social Work* (The Haworth Social Work Practice Press, an imprint of The Haworth Press, Inc.) Vol. 40, No. 1/2, 2002, p. xxi; and: *Older People and Their Caregivers Across the Spectrum of Care* (ed: Judith L. Howe) The Haworth Social Work Practice Press, an imprint of The Haworth Press, Inc., 2003, p. xv. Single or multiple copies of this article are available for a fee from The Haworth Document Delivery Service [1-800-HAWORTH, 9:00 a.m. - 5:00 p.m. (EST). E-mail address: docdelivery@haworthpress.com].

Foreword

The origin of this special volume of the *Journal of Gerontological Social Work* was a videoconference held on June 1, 2001 cosponsored by the Bronx Veterans Affairs Medical Center Geriatric Research Education Clinical Center (GRECC) and the Consortium of New York Geriatric Education Centers (GEC). This videoconference, "Emerging Issues in Social Work & Aging: Revisiting Geriatric Assessment," joined seven Veterans Affairs Medical Centers in New York and New Jersey, drawing over three hundred professionals in a wide range of disciplines from within the VA system and community-based organizations.

This special volume builds on this videoconference. We were particularly interested in topics focusing on geriatric assessment, innovative models of care and caregiving. Suggested foci were "aging in place" strategies, older veterans, cultural diversity, elder abuse, interdisciplinary team approaches, quality of life, mental health, and palliative care. In addition to research-based articles, we sought reports on best practice models. I am very pleased by the quality of the articles contained in this volume.

The keynote address at the videoconference by Barbara Berkman, DSW, Rehr/Fizdale Professor of Social Work at Columbia University, examined the evolution of geriatric assessment over the years and the need to revisit the topic with changes in the health care system, aging patterns, and technology. The ensuing article, by Dr. Berkman, Peter Marimaldi, PhD, CSW, Emily Breon, BA, and myself is included in this volume.

At the conference Dr. Berkman and other professionals in aging, including Gladys Padro-Soler, MPH, Esther Chachkes, DSW, Mathy Mezey, EdD, RN, FANN, and Eileen Chichin, PhD, RN, led an interdisciplinary discussion based on an older woman's progression through the continuum of care: living at home, in a hospital rehabilitation service, and, finally, in a nursing home-based palliative care unit. The title of this special volume,

[Haworth co-indexing entry note]: "Foreword." Howe, Judith L. Co-published simultaneously in *Journal of Gerontological Social Work* (The Haworth Social Work Practice Press, an imprint of The Haworth Press, Inc.) Vol. 40, No. 1/2, 2002, pp. xxiii-xxv; and: *Older People and Their Caregivers Across the Spectrum of Care* (ed: Judith L. Howe) The Haworth Social Work Practice Press, an imprint of The Haworth Press, Inc., 2003, pp. xvii-xix. Single or multiple copies of this article are available for a fee from The Haworth Document Delivery Service [1-800-HAWORTH, 9:00 a.m. - 5:00 p.m. (EST). E-mail address: docdelivery@haworthpress.com].

"Older People and Their Caregivers Across the Spectrum of Care," grew out of this progressive case study. The case focused on the importance of geriatric assessment and reassessment in our work with older people as their situation changes.

It is noteworthy that four of the authors are John A. Hartford Foundation Geriatric Social Work Faculty scholars: Patricia Brownell, CSW, PhD, Letha Chadiha, PhD, Charles Emlet, PhD, MSW, and Michael Parker, LTCR, DSW, PCD, LCSW. Dr. Barbara Berkman, the Principal Investigator of the Hartford Foundation Geriatric Social Work Faculty Scholars Program, deserves great credit for developing this program in concert with the John A. Hartford Foundation and the Gerontological Society of America. They have created a movement which is developing a cadre of leaders in academic geriatric social work. The Scholars Program, now in its third cohort, has had an impressive impact on the fields of social work and gerontology, with a remarkable pace of production and contribution among the Scholars, as evidenced in this special issue.

The issue of caregiving and its intergenerational, financial, and psychosocial implications, is one that needs urgent attention. Just today, I participated in the third and final summit meeting, "Can my Eighties be Like my Fifties?" The New York Academy of Medicine Social Work Fellows, Brookdale Center on Aging/Hunter College, the International Longevity Center-USA, the Bronx VAMC GRECC, Mount Sinai School of Medicine, ARRP, and the Consortium of New York GECs sponsored this conference. This third conference focused on policy and advocacy, with a keynote address by Donna E. Shalala, PhD, President of the University of Miami and former Secretary of the Federal Department of Health and Human Services. John Rother, JD, Policy and Strategy Director for AARP, made responding remarks. This capstone summit built upon the first two summit meetings which focused on the issues facing the Baby Boom generation and educational strategies to prepare Boomers and health professionals for the imminent future. There were many themes that emerged at today's meeting, including the imperative to develop solutions in an intergenerational and community context, particularly the issue of caregiving. It was noted that similar to the advent of the Social Security Program in 1935, caregiving has the potential to propel a social movement with sweeping policy and legislative changes due to its crosscutting and universal nature.

The articles contained in this volume have two dominant threads: *assessment* and *caregiving*. They focus on a myriad of issues related to care across the continuum and the key role of social work assessment in care of the elderly. Dr. Chadiha and her colleagues use a storytelling approach to help African-American women caregivers empower themselves. The vignettes, which were constructed from the caregivers' stories, provide a useful tool for social workers when facilitating woman caregivers' self-empowerment in practice settings. Dr. Dobrof and her colleagues describe the Mount Sinai Medical Center Caregivers and Professional Partnership Program, an interdisciplinary program model aimed at strengthening and sustaining the role and needs of family caregivers of adults. The partnership approach, which encourages caregiver participation, is an exemplar of services geared to older adults and their families. In her paper, Dr. Brownell presents data comparing an elder abuse assessment program providing social services to elder abuse victims with a second program serving elderly victims of crime. She found that both types of programs are effective in serving elder abuse victims. Dr. Emlet and his colleagues discuss the challenges of assessing older adults with HIV/AIDS. This growing and vulnerable population requires sensitive assessment techniques that integrate both geriatric assessment and instruments appropriate for those living with HIV/AIDS. Dr. Corrion and her colleagues report on a secondary analysis of data investigating long-distance caregiving. They conclude that additional research is needed in light of the anticipated future growth of long-distance caregivers and limited knowledge of the patterns and characteristics of support. In his paper, Dr. Parker and his colleagues report on a life course assessment intervention model which is used at the US Army and Air Force Colleges to assist female and male officers to prepare proactively for parent care. They found that the life course model provides a useful framework to guide social workers who help women within and outside the armed forces manage 21st century commitments to family and work. Two articles report on the best practice models. Susan Kornblatt, MA, spotlights the On Lok Program, the prototype of the PACE model of care, and illustrates the benefits of the On Lok model at the end of life of a frail elderly person. Lisa Goodman, ACSW, describes the Northport VA Friendly Companion Program which enhances opportunities for interpersonal interaction, thereby decreasing loneliness, boredom and feelings of isolation. This program was highlighted at a Bronx VAMC GRECC sponsored videoconference on "Quality of Life Issues" held on February 6, 2002.

Sensitive and appropriate assessment is the cornerstone of effective gerontological social work practice. However, as Dr. Berkman and her colleagues state, assessment must be constantly readdressed in light of changes in health care delivery, emergent subpopulations and available technologies for research. It is my hope that this volume captures the importance and complexities of effective assessment and care for older adults and their caregivers in a range of settings and populations.

Judith L. Howe, PhD
October 25, 2002

Social Work Gerontological Assessment Revisited

Barbara J. Berkman, DSW
Peter Maramaldi, PhD, MPH
Emily A. Breon, BA
Judith L. Howe, PhD

SUMMARY. Research has learned much in the last forty years about the factors critical in a gerontological social work assessment. However, assessment must be constantly readdressed, because the context of health care changes and the research technology that enables the study of factors critical to the assessment process becomes more sophisticated.

Barbara J. Berkman is Helen Rehr/Ruth Fizdale Professor of Health and Mental Health, Columbia University School of Social Work. Peter Maramaldi is Assistant Professor at the University of Utah Graduate School of Social Work. Emily A. Breon is affiliated with the Fordham University Law School. Judith L. Howe is Associate Director/Education and Evaluation, GRECC Program, Bronx VAMC; Associate Professor, Brookdale Professor of Geriatrics and Adult Development, Mount Sinai School of Medicine, New York.

Address correspondence to: Barbara Berkman, DSW, Columbia University School of Social Work, 622 West 113th Street, Room 610, New York, NY 10025 (E-mail: bb151@columbia.edu).

Note: This paper is based on the keynote address at the Emerging Issues in Social Work and Aging: Revisiting Geriatric Assessment Videoconference, June 5, 2001 held at the Bronx Veterans Affairs Medical Center, and sponsored by the Bronx VAMC GRECC Program and the Consortium of New York Geriatric Education Centers.

[Haworth co-indexing entry note]: "Social Work Gerontological Assessment Revisited." Berkman, Barbara J. et al. Co-published simultaneously in *Journal of Gerontological Social Work* (The Haworth Social Work Practice Press, an imprint of The Haworth Press, Inc.) Vol. 40, No. 1/2, 2002, pp. 1-14; and: *Older People and Their Caregivers Across the Spectrum of Care* (ed: Judith L. Howe) The Haworth Social Work Practice Press, an imprint of The Haworth Press, Inc., 2003, pp. 1-14. Single or multiple copies of this article are available for a fee from The Haworth Document Delivery Service [1-800-HAWORTH, 9:00 a.m. - 5:00 p.m. (EST). E-mail address: docdelivery@haworthpress.com].

This paper presents the evolution of assessment research and identifies critical assessment factors as related to the changing social work practice in the context of the country's changing health care environment. *[Article copies available for a fee from The Haworth Document Delivery Service: 1-800-HAWORTH. E-mail address: <docdelivery@haworthpress.com> Website: <http://www.HaworthPress.com> © 2002 by The Haworth Press, Inc. All rights reserved.]*

KEYWORDS. Gerontological social work, geriatric assessment, health care, diversity, hospital readmissions, research technology, older cardiac patients, ambulatory care, service needs, psychosocial needs, cultural sensitivity

We have learned much in the last thirty years about the factors critical in a gerontological social work assessment. Assessment should be constantly readdressed because the context of health care changes and the research technology, that allows the study of factors critical to the gerontological assessment process, becomes more sophisticated. With increasingly advanced research available, our knowledge base has grown and there is now the ability to understand and measure, with greater specificity, the key factors needed in assessment.

EARLY ASSESSMENT RESEARCH EFFORTS

The issue of assessment and social work intervention became extremely critical in the late 1960s with the advent of Medicare and Medicaid. Hospital floors were crowded with older patients and the average length of stay of those patients who were helped by social workers was thirty-nine days, compared to eighteen days for patients not referred (Berkman et al., 1971). And, to complicate the situation for social work, patients were referred primarily during the last week of these long stays (Rehr & Gordon, 1967). Social workers needed earlier identification of who, among the increasing numbers of elderly vulnerable inpatients, needed services. The aim of researchers at that time was to isolate factors that would enable early identification and assessment of elderly inpatients that could be helped through social work services. These early research efforts found psychosocial factors to be as important as medical indicators in identifying patients who experienced extended lengths of stay and needed social work help (Berkman & Rehr, 1972). In addition, it was reported that finding patients earlier shortened length of stay (Berkman & Rehr, 1973).

By the 1980s researchers identified the severity and chronicity of illness and level of functioning as critical generic factors in social work assessment (Berkman, Rehr, and Rosenberg, 1980). Study then focused on the identification of disease specific factors. These efforts identified deteriorating mental status and post-hospital stress as significantly related to the elderly cardiac patient's early readmission to the hospital (Berkman & Abrams, 1986). In collaboration with nursing, social workers started to use newly developed standardized measures for research on cardiac patients. Social support was highlighted as a key variable in assessment, and as a major direction for social work intervention to prevent early recurrent admissions (Berkman et al., 1987).

In the 1990s, again in collaboration with nursing, social work researchers explored assessment factors which were useful in predicting who, among cardiac patients, were at risk for early readmission because of functional, psychological, social and environmental problems (Berkman et al., 1990, 1991). The most significant findings from that series of studies was that when social work services in the initial admission were limited to information and referral only, without assessment, that these patients would again need help from social workers upon readmission. And, if a social work assessment was conducted during the first admission and potential barriers to the *completion* of the post-hospital discharge plan were identified, but not addressed, that these patients would again need social work help upon readmission.

CURRENT CONTEXT OF HEALTHCARE AND ASSESSMENT PRACTICES

It is important to understand the context of health care in which we are now engaged in assessment. Traditionally, our health care system has been based on a paradigm of unpredictable acute disease; this model has become somewhat inappropriate. Technological advances in technology and science have enabled significantly fewer hospitalizations and reduced patient length of stay. Increasing numbers of elder patients are presenting in ambulatory settings with multiple, chronic health problems. These patients are living in the community with frailty and are increasingly at risk of losing their ability to function independently (Berkman, 1996).

In the new health care paradigm characterized by chronic illness, episodes of need for care can be more predictable (Pawlson, 1994), and there is awareness that chronic illnesses and their progression are determined by many factors, such as an individual's social, psychological, and physical environment and genetic endowment, along with health care accessibility factors (Evans, 1994; Syme, 1994). Thus we find an increasing focus on primary care with disease prevention and health promotion our significant interest (Pawlson, 1994). The vulnerable chronically ill elderly, traditionally the major focus of social work services, present complex interacting medical and psychosocial problems associated with aging. Screening for those at risk for physical, social, or psychological regression, and assessment of their needs, becomes much more essential in this new model, and the timing of intervention by health care professionals remains paramount (Berkman, 1996).

Thus, an important aspect of our health care context is that the acute care model of care, long the focus of geriatric social work in hospitals, is no longer sufficient because of the needs of the chronically ill older population for continuity of care and not just episodic interventions. The elderly person who has chronic care needs may require rehabilitation and a range of supportive services from home care to meal preparations, to counseling, to adult day care, to respite care, to acute and long term care. Health care is beginning to respond to the increasing needs for continuity of care through creation of community-based networks linking service providers to a continuum of health care services (Berkman & Volland, 1997).

Social workers can now be found working in every site providing health and mental health services to the elderly (Berkman et al., 1997). They help older people who are active and healthy, as well as those who have poor health, and address the needs of the elderly who live in the community, as well as those hospitalized or in long term care institutions. Traditional sites for social work practice include: hospitals and ambulatory care clinics; community mental health centers, family services, and community long term care settings which include nursing homes, home health and homemaker service agencies. In addition, we have adult day care, rehabilitation centers and other service agencies for elder care. More recently, social workers are helping the elderly and their families in: independent physician practices; dental clinics; managed care companies; and corporations which offer employee assistance programs, elder care or dependent care programs. Regardless of site, regardless of role, screening and assessment of need for psychosocial help is still the most important part of service delivery and is the beginning of the intervention process.

Thus, social workers have the opportunity to serve the aging population and their families through the continuum of care based on predetermined vulnerable points in a chronic illness. Therefore, the focus of social work research has begun to move out of hospital inpatient services and into community ambulatory sites but with what is basically a revisit to the first gerontological assessment research question "Who needs social work services and what do they need?" (Berkman et al., 1999). With increasing numbers of elderly with chronic illness living in the community, screening and assessment becomes increasingly important to the provision of continuity of care to identify those with biopsychosocial needs. Many people are not aware of available social services and families with serious social problems are not finding the community resources and services they need. Thus, in the context of the changing health care environment, we must constantly readdress our approaches to assessment and identify its critical components.

Social workers emphasize the biopsychosocial focus to assessing the needs of older individuals and families (Berkman & Volland, 1997). This focus, within a multidisciplinary collaborative approach to care, can provide social work a major place within emerging health delivery systems. Our biopsychosocial approach gives social workers a carefully balanced perspective that takes into account the entire person in his or her environment, and helps in the assessment of the needs of an individual from a multidimensional point of view. The need to understand what are the critical assessment factors is going to be increasingly important in health planning and clinical practice to determine treatment and rehabilitation needs along the continuum of service delivery.

The demand for social work service in geriatrics will be increasing well into the next century. The focus of the biopsychosocial geriatric social work assessment is on physical, psychological, social and environmental factors that create or contribute to problems in living. However, social work assessment also focuses on the older person's strengths and adaptive capacities, with the goal of alleviating and/or preventing problems. In this assessment, we understand the importance of the informal caregiving network; the older person's significant relationships and the emotional and financial stresses of caregivers are recognized. Social workers can then utilize knowledge of formal support systems (for example, home health care or senior centers) and entitlements, such as

Medicare and Social Security, to help the elderly and their caregivers obtain needed supportive resources.

This professional perspective, which integrates multiple systems, enables social workers to understand the interaction among factors that have an effect on the way the elderly person responds to illness, disability, and the health care system, bringing a unique and necessary dimension to the multidisciplinary approach that is so important to the field of geriatrics. If psychosocial needs go unmet through misdiagnosis, lack of detection, lack of treatment and follow up, elderly patients are at risk of further health problems that can lead to physical deterioration, reduced independence, and eventually to the need for more intensive and expensive services (Shearer, Simmons, White, & Berkman, 1995). Inadequate assessment also can lead to inappropriate long-term care and unnecessary institutional placements. Medical management of the frail elderly patient requires a comprehensive approach that includes careful assessment of complex medical problems and functional capabilities, social supports, and emotional well being.

WHY NOT JUST STANDARDIZED ASSESSMENT MEASURES?

Social work assessment is key to intervention, but not just for the information obtained. If it were merely this social work could rely totally on the many standardized measures available for assessing geriatric depression, dementia, quality of life, physical functioning, ADL functioning and IADL functioning, to name a few. These standardized tools may give beginning clues that a person needs help but will not clarify the direction of help.

Standardized measures are valuable in screening for those who need further assessment but should not be the definitive assessment. Rather, these reliable and valid measures give us data we can use in assessment and allows us to uniformly compare groups of patients. The assessment itself is an integral part of the professional intervention as part of the clinical process. Through direct discussion with the client and important others in the clients' intervention network, the process enables the social worker to understand the client's typical behavior, coping capacities, motivations, and the nature of relationships. In addition, we can discover the social environmental resources that are both needed and acceptable and find out what resources are available.

How the client and social worker interact during assessment may be your best clue as to how the older person interacts with others. Assessment gives us the knowledge we need to develop an individualized plan and may have clinical value as the start of a trusting relationship with the client and family. While there are available multidimensional assessment measures used to evaluate the elderly clients' circumstances and capabilities, these instruments are frequently long and complex and will not assess critical interrelationship issues that are so important for a plan of action.

Assessment by case managers and other staff in long-term care has its own particular issues for here comprehensive measurement tools frequently are used to determine the needs of clients for health and social services and financial eligibility for those services. However, these assessment methods, while attempting to achieve uniform decision making, have been criticized for faulty administration and poor judgements that are made on the basis of the data (Geron, 1997).

Effective assessment requires specialized skills, such as: interviewing techniques, empathy, knowledge of human behavior, and of family and caregiver dynamics (Geron & Chassler, 1994). Long-term care decisions should involve choices that ideally are made by clients with the help of an expert (Kane & Degenholtz, 1997). The difficult questions are how do we assess the values of an individual's preferences? This is not done consistently when we use current long-term care assessment measurement tools. As Scott Geron (1997) has said, what we need are assessment protocols which clearly "enhance clinical decision-making and facilitate professional judgement" (p. 7). Ideally, standardized assessments should enhance and facilitate the process of the clinical interview. The judgement of the interviewer is critical, for it is this skilled clinician who must know when to follow-up on questions and when the clients' concerns must be addressed.

CULTURALLY SENSITIVE ASSESSMENT NEEDED

Particularly troubling is that there is a lack of culturally sensitive assessment protocols. A major demographic trend impacting health care services is the increased social and ethnic diversity of the elder population. Before the middle of the next century, the non-white ethnic minorities such as African Americans, American Indian/Alaska Natives, Asian/Pacific Island Americans and Hispanic Americans are projected to make up twenty percent of all older Americans (Berkman et al., 2000). There are vast differences culturally in factors affecting our assessment of older adults in terms of health beliefs, health care utilization, health risks, and patterns of relationships with family members. And even within ethnic groups there is vast diversity.

In addition, the older population includes other groups that require specific knowledge, sensitivity and interventions. These groups include persons with alternate lifestyles (such as gay or lesbian persons, persons whose religious beliefs vary significantly from our majority culture, and persons with developmental disabilities). Finally, there are those elderly with special needs who have diseases, illnesses, or face social problems which often carry large amounts of shame and stigma from society, such as persons suffering from HIV/AIDS, alcoholism, drug addiction, and mental illness (Berkman et al., 2000). Emotional reactions of the elderly, related to physical health issues, are interrelated with personal and culturally bound perceptions which influence their access to, acceptance of, and utilization of health care services. The extraordinary diversity of this population creates complex problems in the assessment of needs for heath and social services. Social work service delivery must be especially cognizant of the cultural diversity among elders who confront serious physical and mental health problems.

Another factor increasing diversity among our older population is the defined "older" age period that can now span several generations. The knowledge base needed by geriatric social workers to conduct an assessment includes understanding the differences in the psychosocial challenges faced by 65 year olds and those who are 85 years old, who are in very different stages of their life cycles. And, in fact, in many situations the sixty-five year old is the caregiver for an older parent.

We must commit to developing culturally sensitive approaches to service, including assessment. Culture challenges us as assessors to consider not only the cultural diversity among our clients, but we must consider our own cultural assumptions in order to understand how this affects our expectations of the client (Yee, 1997). Practitioners and clients often come from different cultural backgrounds and may not share the same perception of illness or expectations for health care (Kramer, 2001). Finally, cultural competence cannot focus only on language, but involves body language such as eye contact and touching, which also may be important (Mackenzie, 2000). Thus, when we consider the multitude of factors related to cultural diversity, such as age differentials, acculturation levels, primary language, education level, race or ethnicity, and religion, we understand the challenges we face in achieving culturally sensitive and valued assessment (Mackenzie, 2000).

MAJOR FACTORS IN ASSESSMENT

There are several specific major factors identified that must be considered in a social work gerontological assessment.

Functional problems: The critical importance of functional disability which is associated with severe and chronic illness and which frequently increases with age cannot be emphasized enough. Stroke, arthritis, hip fracture, congestive heart failure, and chronic pulmonary disease–such as emphysema–are associated with mobility problems, generalized weaknesses, and an inability to perform both basic and instrumental activities of daily living. Functional disability may be the result of interacting physical problems, such as negative effects of treatment and medication interactive effects, dementing illnesses, such as Alzheimer's, and their associated cognitive loss also lead to functional disability, as can emotional problems. Services that compensate for such impairments tend to be labor intensive and expensive. Receiving such services requires many social and psychological adjustments for older people and their families. There may be a decrease in resources and in the availability of family assistance. These problems, in conjunction with illness and increased dependency, can lead to increases in the admissions of the elderly to hospitals and long-term care. The need for social work assessment of functionally related psychosocial needs is paramount to successful service delivery.

Key factors, such as functioning, have many determinants involving a combination of interacting psychological, physical, social and cultural factors. It is clear that the geriatric assessment of the elderly may need the input of many health professionals. In some settings this is relatively natural, but now in community settings, the autonomous social worker may need to take a broader role in getting the data needed in undertaking a valid assessment.

Psychological Problems: Psychological factors can interact with functional capacity to exacerbate the severity of many illnesses, general disability, and recovery. It is not unusual for an individual to react with depression, anxiety and denial when experiencing a major illness. These three psychological factors have been identified as relating to problems in the recovery of elderly patients. The challenge for social workers in assessment is to disentangle the causes of impairment and alleviate that amenable to treatment.

Cognitive Problems: The number of people with cognitive impairment has increased dramatically as the older population increases (U.S. Bureau of the Census, 1993). Cognitive problems present significant issues for quality of life of the elderly and caregivers (Freed, Elder, Lauderdale, & Carter, 1999). Quality of life (QoL) is a multidimensional concept concerning social, psychological, and physical factors (Birren, Lubben, & Rowe, 1991). Heath care providers can intervene and affect QoL for individuals with dementia even though we may not be able to change the course of the disease (Brod, Stewart, Sands & Walton, 1999). A person's QoL is a subjective, individual experience (Callahan, 1992). Dementia patients, regardless of the similarities of their conditions, may have very different QoL because of different attitudes, beliefs and circumstances and can be considered good informants of their own subjective states (Brod, Stewart, Sands, & Walton, 1999). Dementia has incredible consequences both financially and emotionally for patients and families (Schulz, O'Brien, Bookwala, & Fleissner, 1995). The initial assessment must be thorough and accurate because of its primary importance as the basis for appropriate planning (Freed, Elder, Lauderdale, & Carter, 1999; Chodosh, 2001).

Social Support Problems: An emerging social trend is that families are increasingly expected to be responsible for the home care needs of their loved ones. With the number of beneficiaries of the Medicare Home Health program rising significantly each year, this pressure on families has been increasing (U. S. Special Committee on Aging, 1996). However, families may not have the physical, psychological or financial resources needed to provide such care (Berkman & Volland, 1997). The capacity of families to adapt to the patient's medical condition has led to a renewed focus on family assessment and therapy (Glassman, 1991).

Social support encompasses emotional support, advice, and guidance, as well as the material aid and services that people obtain from their social relationships. Social support has been found to maximize adaptation and coping and also enhances self-esteem and self-control. Maintaining social networks has been found to be related to lower rates of hospital admission and readmission and to be beneficial to recovery. Lack of social support and feelings of loneliness have been correlated with illness, disability, and higher mortality rates (Abrams, Beers, & Berkow, 1995).

However, not all social support has positive effects. Excessive family attention may lead to greater disability, either by family members' doing too much for the geriatric patient or by their verbally discouraging activity. In addition, the long term care of a chronically ill family member may result in too many expectations placed on the caregivers. As the situation grows less tolerable, and the strain increases with the chronicity of the illness, the caregivers may distance themselves, and the elderly may experience an increase in feelings of loneliness. Assessment of social support is absolutely essential. Social workers must consider both the elderly person's biopsychosocial needs and the family's adapting and coping capacity.

Grief and Loss Problems: Older people suffer from many losses at a stage in life when physiological reserves are at their lowest. Such losses may be conceptualized in four categories: the aging process; health; death of others; and social and environmental losses, such as loss of income, meaningful and productive social roles and activities, with the possible resultant loss of status, respect and self-esteem. This is an important dimension for assessment as social work can play a significant role in helping the older person cope with late life losses and stresses.

Hospitalization Related Problems: The elderly admitted to hospitals are generally in need of acute treatment for multiple conditions. Admission to the hospital takes its toll physiological and psychologically on elderly and their families. Elders who experience the disruption of a hospitalization may also have heightened fears of increased dependency on family members. It is understandable that they may react to being hospitalized with anxiety and fear, which cause additional stress on their physiological system. These stressors increase the risk of the patient's becoming confused and disoriented and therefore less able to manage the postdischarge care necessitated by the illness.

When the patient's capacity to comply with medical recommendations is compromised, the likelihood of a readmission to the hospital increases. These patients are considered "high risk" individuals who need assessment and service from social workers in making the transition from the hospital to posthospital care, whether to their own homes or to other facilities. Moreover, with even shorter hospital stays and the tendency to discharge older people for brief recuperative stays in nursing homes, short-term nursing home residents need extra social work services. Social workers, sometimes bearing the title of *case manager*, have been called on to conduct comprehensive assessments of the older person's physical, psychological, cognitive, and social functioning and to allocate home care according to a care plan that is acceptable to the older person and the family while carefully weighing the risks and benefits of home care in their recommendations.

Abuse Problems: Although abuse of older people has been recognized as a distinct social issue only since the late 1970s, all states now have some programs to detect and treat this problem. It should be noted that neglect is the leading type of abuse, followed by physical abuse.

The third most common form of abuse is financial and material exploitation, which includes such actions as taking or using the property of the older person without permission, appropriating pension and social security funds, and otherwise misusing the older adult's resources. The majority of abusers are relatives; adult children, spouses and others. A greater proportion of older women than older men is abused. Social work assessment of the possibility of abuse and neglect is critical.

End of Life Issues: All social workers practicing in health care have an important function in palliative and end-of-life care when they are increasingly called on to assist older people and their family members in clarifying the alternatives in achieving comfort with their treatment decisions. They are the most frequently identified professionals to provide emotional counseling services, and they provide support, communication, assistive services and advocacy to the families of the ill patient. An assessment must be made to determine whether patients and caregivers are willing to discuss end-of-life care decisions. In this assessment, clinicians must be informed on the patient's and family's understanding of the situation which includes the biological, psychological, and social situation in addition to spiritual issues associated with dying and beliefs about death held by the patient and significant others. These vary significantly due to cultural experiences (Kramer, 2001).

Elderly persons with chronic diseases and activity limitation represent an increasing percentage of all persons served by social workers and the health care system. The goal of health care for the elderly cannot be just to provide "good medicine" or "good nursing" but rather must focus on how the patient can manage his or her health optimally to enhance quality of life. The growing number of elderly with chronic disabling illnesses, and the increasing need for biopsychosocial rehabilitative services to support independent functioning, means that patients and families will require more psychosocial assistance in order to address their health care problems effectively (Browne et al., 1996). Social workers and other health professionals trained in gerontology will become even more essential in health care to assess and address the complex needs of older people and their families.

REFERENCES

Abrams, W., Beers, M., & Berkow, R. (Eds.). (1995). *The Merck Manual of Geriatrics* (p. 1401). Whitehouse Station, NJ: Merck & Company, Inc.

Berkman, B., Silverstone, B., Simmons, W. J., Howe, J., & Volland, P. (2000). Social work gerontological practice: The need for faculty development in the new millennium. *Journal of Gerontological Social Work, 34* (1), 5-23.

Berkman, B., Chauncey, S., Holmes, W., Daniels, A., Bonander, E., Sampson, S., & Robinson, M. (1999). Standardized screening of older patients' needs for social work assessment in primary care: Use of the SF 36. *Health and Social Work, 24* (1), 1-80.

Berkman, B., Dobrof, R., Harry, L., & Damron-Rodriguez, J. (1997). Social work. In S. M. Klein (Ed.), *A natural agenda for geriatric education: White papers* (pp. 53-85). New York: Springer.

Berkman, B., & Volland, P. (1997). Health care practice overview. In R. L. Edwards (Ed.), *Encyclopedia of social work, 19th edition* (pp. 143-149). Washington, DC: NASW Press.

Berkman, B. (1996). The emerging health care world: Implications for social work practice and education. *Social Work, 41* (5), 541-551.

Berkman, B., Millar, S., Holmes, W., & Bonander, E. (1991). Predicting elderly cardiac patients at risk for readmission. *Social Work in Health Care, 16* (1), 21-38.

Berkman, B., Millar, S., Holmes, W., & Bonander, E. (1990). Screening elder cardiac patients to identify need for social work services. *Health and Social Work,* 15(1): 64-72.

Berkman, B., Dumas, S., Gastfriend, J., Poplawski, J., & Southworth, M. (1987). Predicting hospital readmission of elderly cardiac patients. *Health and Social Work, 12* (3), 221-228.

Berkman, B., & Abrams, R. (1986). Factors related to early readmission of elderly cardiac patients. *Social Work, 31* (2), 99-103.

Berkman, B., Rehr, H., & Rosenberg, G. (1980). A social work department develops and tests a screening mechanism to identify high social risk situations. *Social Work in Health Care, 5* (4), 373-386.

Berkman, B., & Rehr, H. (1973). Early social service casefinding for hospital patients: An experiment. *Social Service Review, 47* (2), 256-265.

Berkman, B., & Rehr, H. (1972). The "sick role" cycle and the timing of social work intervention. *Social Service Review, 46* (4), 567-580.

Berkman, B., Rehr, H., Siegel, D., Paneth, J., & Pomrinse, S. D. (1971). Utilization of inpatient services by the elderly. *Journal of the American Geriatrics Society, 19* (11), 933-946.

Birren, J., Lubben, J., & Rowe, J. (1991). *The concept of measurement of quality of life in the frail elderly.* San Diego, CA: Academic Press.

Brod, M., Stewart, A. L., Sands, L., & Walton, P. (1999). Conceptualization and measurement of quality of life in dementia: The dementia quality of life instrument (DqoL). *The Gerontologist, 39* (1), 25-35.

Browne, C. V., Smith, M., & Ewalt, P. L. (1996). Advancing social work practice in health care settings: A collaborative partnership for continuing education. *Health and Social Work, 21* (4), 267-276.

Callahan, S. (1992). Ethics and dementia: Current issues . . . quality of life. *Alzheimer Disease and Associated Disorders, 6* (3). 138-144.

Chodosh, J. (2001). Cognitive screening tests: The mini-mental status exam. In M. D. Mezey (Ed.), *The encyclopedia of elder care* (pp. 142-144). New York: Springer.

Evans, R. C. (1994). Health care as a threat to health: Defense, opulence, and the social environment. *Health and Wealth, 123* (4), 21-42.

Freed, D. M., Elder, W., Lauderdale, S., & Carter, S. (1999). An integrated program for dementia evaluation and care management. *The Gerontologist, 39* (3), 356-361.

Geron, S. M. (1997). Multidimensional assessment measures. Generations: *Journal of the American Society on Aging, 21* (1), 52-54.

Geron, S. M., & Chassler, D. (1994). Guidelines for case management practice across long-term care continuum. *Report of the National Advisory Committee on Long-Term Care Case Management.* Bristol, CT: Connecticut Community Care, Inc.

Glassman, U. (1991). The social work group and its distinct qualities in the health care setting. *Health and Social Work, 16* (3), 203-212.

Kane, R. A., & Degenholtz, H. (1997). Assessing values and preferences: Should we, can we? *Generations: Journal of the American Society on Aging, 21* (1), 19-24.

Kramer, B. J. (2001). Cultural assessment. In M. D. Mezey (Ed.), *The encyclopedia of elder care* (pp. 116-119). New York: Springer.

Mackenzie, E. R. (2000). Cultural competence increases healthcare access for at-risk elders. *Healthcare and Aging, 7* (3), 1-6.

Pawlson, L. G. (1994). Chronic illness: Implications of a new paradigm for health care. *Joint Commission Journal on Quality Improvement, 20* (1), 33-39.

Rehr, H., & Gordon, B. (1967). Aging ward patients and the hospital social service department. *Journal of American Geriatrics Society, 25* (12), 1153-1162.

Schulz, R., O'Brien, A. T., Bookwala, J., & Fleissner, K. (1995). Psychiatric and physical morbidity effects of dementia caregiving: Prevalence, correlates, and causes. *The Gerontologist, 35,* 771-791.

Shearer, S., Simmons, J., White, M., & Berkman, B. (1995). Physician partnership project: Social work case management in primary care. *Continuum: An interdisciplinary journal on continuity of care,* July/August, 1-7.

Syme, S. L. (1994). The social environment and health. *Health and Wealth, 123* (4), 79-86.

U.S. Bureau of the Census. (1993). Sixty-five plus in America. In C. Taeuber (Ed.), *Current population reports (Series P-23-178RV).* Washington, DC: U.S. Government Printing Office.

U. S. Special Committee on Aging. (1996). *GAO report to the Chairman.* Washington, DC: Author.

Yee, D. (1997). Can long-term care assessments be culturally responsive? *Generations: Journal of the American Society on Aging, 21* (1), 25-29.

Best Practice:
The On Lok Model
of Geriatric Interdisciplinary Team Care

Susan Kornblatt, MA
Sabrina Cheng, MSW
Susana Chan, MSW

SUMMARY. On Lok Senior Health Services provides community-based comprehensive care for the frail elderly and is the prototype of the PACE (Program of All-Inclusive Care for the Elderly) model of care. Comprehensive care includes all aspects of acute care and long term care under one capitated health delivery system. The cornerstone of care at On Lok is the interdisciplinary team that performs a comprehensive assessment of all participants at intake and at regular intervals after enrollment. The team consists of physician, social worker, nurse, physical therapist, occupational therapist, dietitian, home care nurse, geriatric aide, driver, recreation therapist and other specialists as needed. The team uses standardized instruments, develops treatment plans for each participant and meets at least four times per week to discuss cases. The case presented illustrates the benefits of the On

---

Susan Kornblatt is Director of Education and Training at On Lok, Inc., San Francisco. Sabrina Cheng and Susana Chan, MSW, are both social workers, On Lok Senior Health Services.

[Haworth co-indexing entry note]: "Best Practice: The On Lok Model of Geriatric Interdisciplinary Team Care." Kornblatt, Susan, Sabrina Cheng, and Susana Chan. Co-published simultaneously in *Journal of Gerontological Social Work* (The Haworth Social Work Practice Press, an imprint of The Haworth Press, Inc.) Vol. 40, No. 1/2, 2002, pp. 15-22; and: *Older People and Their Caregivers Across the Spectrum of Care* (ed: Judith L. Howe) The Haworth Social Work Practice Press, an imprint of The Haworth Press, Inc., 2003, pp. 15-22. Single or multiple copies of this article are available for a fee from The Haworth Document Delivery Service [1-800-HAWORTH, 9:00 a.m. - 5:00 p.m. (EST). E-mail address: docdelivery@haworthpress.com].

Lok model of interdisciplinary care through the end of life of a frail elderly person. *[Article copies available for a fee from The Haworth Document Delivery Service: 1-800-HAWORTH. E-mail address: <docdelivery@haworthpress.com> Website: <http://www.HaworthPress.com> © 2002 by The Haworth Press, Inc. All rights reserved.]*

KEYWORDS. Geriatric interdisciplinary team care, comprehensive geriatric assessment, interdisciplinary team assessment, comfort care, PACE, On Lok, team treatment planning, standardized instruments, team goals, discipline-specific goals

INTRODUCTION

On Lok Senior Health Services provides community-based comprehensive medical, social and rehabilitative services to frail elderly persons in San Francisco and Fremont, California. Currently On Lok has 905 enrollees, each of whom is assigned to a team at one of On Lok's eight centers. On Lok integrates acute care and long term care under one health delivery system with service revenues provided through capitation payments from Medicare, Medicaid and private payments. Funds from these sources are combined into an unrestricted pool to pay for all health and related services provided to On Lok enrollees. Capitated reimbursement requires the assessment of risk and strategic use of resources. While On Lok as an organization assumes full financial risk for the care of all enrollees, health care providers and health care teams are not responsible to track individual costs of care for those patients (Kornblatt, Eng, and O'Malley, 2001).

On Lok is the prototype for PACE, the Program of All-Inclusive Care for the Elderly (Eng et al., 1997). Currently 35 PACE sites in the United States serve over 8350 frail elderly persons (National PACE Association, 2001). PACE provides all care for enrollees including primary care, social work, restorative therapy, home care and institutional care in both hospital and nursing home settings. Specialty and ancillary medical services are also provided, as are long term care services including transportation, meals and personal care. Since fixed, per capita payments cover all care, enrollees pay no additional copayments or other fees. Participants of On Lok must use the On Lok team of care providers and contracted specialists, hospitals and nursing homes.

GERIATRIC INTERDISCIPLINARY TEAM ASSESSMENT

Comprehensive geriatric assessment is widely viewed as the most effective way of addressing the multiple interrelated needs of the frail elderly. Geriatric assessment is the multidimensional process designed to assess an elderly person's functional ability (Boult, 2000). Interdisciplinary geriatric assessment and care can be more effective than professionals working alone (Fulmer and Hyer, 2000). The cornerstone of care at On Lok, and all the PACE programs, is the geriatric interdisciplinary team. The team manages care through direct service provision, continuous patient assessment, treatment planning, coordination of contract services, and monitoring of quality of care (Eng, 1996). Freed from the constraints of fee-for-service payment systems, teams have great flexibility in decision-making.

A comprehensive interdisciplinary team assessment is performed on every On Lok enrollee at intake. This evaluation includes an assessment of four key domains:

- Physical health and medical conditions
- Functional ability and status
- Cognitive and mental health
- Psychosocial function/socioenvironmental situation

At intake the primary care practitioner (physician or nurse practitioner), nurse, social worker, physical therapist, occupational therapist, dietitian and home care nurse conduct in-person assessments of the participant's health and functional status. This assessment includes detailed information regarding:

- *Medical history*: current conditions, past hospitalizations, surgery, current medications, immunizations, tobacco use, alcohol use and other relevant information.
- *Physical exam*: blood pressure, cardiovascular, musculoskeletal and neurologic information.
- *Social history*: living arrangements, formal and informal caregivers, monthly income, significant life history, capacity to cope.
- *Functional assessment*: activities of daily living and instrumental activities of daily living.
- *Home assessment*: access to home, such as stairs and elevator; safety in the kitchen, bedroom and bathroom; adequacy of meal

preparation; compliance to medication regimen; evidence of alcohol abuse.

Each discipline contributes its special skills to assess each element. For example, medical conditions are assessed by the physician/nurse practitioner; the nurse, occupational therapist, physical therapist and dietitian all evaluate aspects of the participant's functional status; medication use is assessed by the nurse; the social worker helps to evaluate cognition (memory, orientation, reasoning and attention span), mood and behavior (affect, depression, anxiety, fear and thought disorder); the social worker also conducts individual and family interviews to assess enrollees' psycho-social history which includes aspects of coping skills, housing needs and support systems. Ability to cook and bathe is assessed by the occupational therapist; ability to transfer is assessed by the physical therapist and ability to feed oneself is assessed by the dietitian and occupational therapist. The occupational therapist examines functional status, ability to perform ADLs such as dressing, grooming and feeding, as well as the Independent Activities of Daily Living (IADLs) such as shopping and chores. The occupational therapist also gathers information about safety of the home. The Home Care Registered Nurse (HCRN) interviews the applicant and the family regarding the applicant's ability to provide self care and hygiene and/or the family's ability to continue support in those areas. Three other disciplines, physical therapy, nutrition and recreation administer their evaluation within one week of the participant's enrollment.

The team uses standardized instruments to evaluate cognition, function and affect. These include: Mini Mental Status Exam (Folstein et al., 1975), Short Portable Mental Status Questionnaire (Pfeiffer, 1975), Activities of Daily Living Index (Katz et al., 1963), Instrumental Activities of Daily Living scales (Lawton and Brody, 1969), Geriatric Depression Scale (Yesavage et al., 1983) and Tinetti Balance and Gait Scale (1986). After conducting their individual assessments and identifying interventions, team members develop a comprehensive treatment plan. This plan addresses the four key domains of the interdisciplinary geriatric assessment and includes some team goals and some discipline-specific goals, with interventions that may involve one or more disciplines for each of the goals.

Every On Lok interdisciplinary team meets formally a minimum of four times per week to update, review and discuss participant conditions. Members of the team also meet together to discuss specific participant changes on an as-needed basis. Medically stable participants undergo a complete re-assessment with a formal review of their individual care plans by the entire interdisciplinary team, every three to six months. Acute situations are handled by the team daily.

Case Study: Mrs. Y

Mrs. Y was born in Hong Kong. As a widow, she immigrated to San Francisco in 1991 with five of her seven adult children. She enrolled in On Lok SeniorHealth (OLSH) in 1995 after suffering a stroke, a right-sided CVA with left-sided hemiparesis. The OLSH interdisciplinary team assessed and evaluated Mrs. Y, identifying 15 medical problems. Her two primary diagnoses were congestive heart failure (CHF) and diabetes mellitus, type one (DM1).

Upon enrollment, Mrs. Y lived at home with one of her daughters, who was the primary caregiver. Consistent with On Lok's efforts to partner with families in providing comprehensive care, Mrs. Y's family was committed to this partnership. Her children and grandchildren visited frequently and were very attentive to her needs. Mrs. Y's care plan included a combination of OLSH services: visits to the adult day health center, a good nutrition program, frequent follow-up care in the medical clinic, a maintenance physical therapy program and home care assistance from On Lok as needed.

As often occurs, family dynamics were sometimes difficult and the siblings argued amongst themselves about the care plan for their mother. The OLSH social worker facilitated regular family conferences to assist in the health care decision-making process. The primary care nurse practitioner and other members of the interdisciplinary team participated regularly to provide education and consultation. With the support of the social worker and her daughter, Mrs. Y was able to state her preferences for care very clearly and all of her children were respectful of her wishes.

In her seventh year under the care of On Lok, Mrs. Y's CHF condition worsened and her edema could no longer be controlled by medication or any alternative means. The cardiologist evaluated her and explained to her and to her family that there were no treatments available. Although the concept of "comfort care" had been described to her family members previously, when the time came for further exploring this option, her family needed more information and support. The physician and the social worker coordinated a family conference to address family concerns and answer questions. They explained that comfort care is an active and holistic treatment to enhance quality of life once rescue or life-sustaining medical interventions are no longer desired or beneficial. They helped the family understand that efforts to ensure comfort and well-being of the patient and family were not "giving up" or "doing nothing" (Stinson & Laguna Honda Hospital Bioethics Committee, 1997). On Lok staff described comfort care as treatment, such as pain control, directed at physical symptoms, along with emotional and psychosocial support, needed for spiritual distress. Several family members stated that their wish was to have Mrs. Y die at home, but the daughter who was Mrs. Y's primary caregiver objected. She felt she could no longer manage the heavy care required. On Lok staff helped the family understand that their mother's heart condition was irreversible and that her daily care required difficult transfers and round-the-clock supervision.

Because Mrs. Y remained alert and oriented, she was able to convince her family that she would be more comfortable staying in one of On Lok's housing buildings instead of her home. She chose to stay in the hospice room at On Lok House, which is designed to provide comfort care for On Lok participants during their final days and weeks. On Lok House has 70 HUD-supported residential units and its lower floors house one of the On Lok SeniorHealth clinics and day health centers. Thus housing, health and social services are all located in one building. Once unit with four beds is set aside for hospice when needed by On Lok participants. Mrs. Y spent her final days either in her room at On Lok House or in the day health center. She managed to go to the center daily for breakfast, to receive her morning medication, to meet her friends, to be examined by medical staff and to receive personal care with assistance of geriatric aides, who checked her around the clock. Mrs. Y completed her life in the care of the interdisciplinary team and her family. The physician or nurse practitioner visited her daily to check her vital signs, her skin, heart and edema. Nearing the ultimate part of her life, when she could no longer attend the day health center, the staff turned her in her bed when she was unable to do so herself. The social worker made daily visits to Mrs. Y to provide psychosocial and emotional support to Mrs. Y and her family. Spiritual support in the form of Bible reading, praying and hymn singing by a church group was arranged and provided at Mrs. Y's request. Although Mrs. Y's medical conditions could not be reversed, the On Lok team was committed to making her feel comfortable and provided oxygen and pain medication as needed. Her family, also dedicated to her care, provided additional companionship and emotional support. Her children visited every day, bringing her favorite homemade foods and reading and singing to her. Mrs. Y's children joined her in the day health center while she was still able to get there, or had more intimate contact with Mrs. Y in the privacy of her room.

Mrs. Y died after three months of comfort care. The family came to accept the team's recommendation for comfort care and appreciated the peace of mind that came with On Lok's commitment to provide optimum care. The comfort care plan helped alleviate stress on the family and provided confidence that their mother was in capable hands. Just after she died, Mrs. Y's family invited all of the On Lok staff who cared for her to enjoy a fellowship luncheon, a meaningful Chinese tradition and expression of appreciation after the end of life. All of those who were involved in her care attended and were joined by her family members. This case illustrates the spirit of "On Lok," which in Chinese means "peaceful and happy abode" and it also demonstrates the benefits to older persons and their families of the interdisciplinary team approach to care.

REFERENCES

Boult, C. (2000). Comprehensive Geriatric Assessment. In The Merck Manual of Geriatrics, 3rd. edition. Eds. Beers, M., and Berkow, R. Merck & Co., Inc.

Eng, C., Pedulla, J., Eleazar, P., McCann, R., and Fox, N. (1997). Program of all-inclusive care for the elderly (PACE): An innovative model of integrated geriatric care and financing. Journal of the American Geriatrics Society. 45:223-232.

Eng, C. (1996). The On Lok/PACE model of geriatric managed care: an interdisciplinary approach to care of the frail elderly. Current Concepts in Geriatric Managed Care. Vol. 2, No. 9: 4-24.

Folstein, M., Folstein, S., and McHugh, P. (1975). Mini-Mental State: A practical method for grading the cognitive state of patients for the clinician. Journal of Psychiatric Research, Vol 12: 189-198.

Fulmer, T., and Hyer, K. (2000). Geriatric Interdisciplinary Teams. In The Merck Manual of Geriatrics, 3rd. edition. Eds. Beers, M., and Berkow, R. Merck & Co., Inc.

Katz et al. (1963). Katz Index of Activities of Daily Living. Journal of the American Medical Association. Vol 185: 914-919.

Kornblatt, S., O'Malley, K., and Eng, C. (2002). Refusing to comply: What do you do when the interdisciplinary team plan doesn't work? In Ethical Patient Care: A Casebook for Geriatric Health Care Teams, Mezey et. al, eds. Johns Hopkins Press.

Lawton, M., and Brody, E. (1969). Assessment of Older People: Self Maintaining and Instrumental Activities of Daily Living. The Gerontologist. Vol 9: 179-186.

National PACE Association (2001). January-June 2001 PACE Cross-Site Comparison Report. June 2001.

Pfeiffer, E. (1975). Short Portable Mental Status Questionnaire (SPMSQ). In Israel, L, Kozarevic, D., and Sartorius, N. (1984). Source book of geriatric assessment. (2 vols). Vol. 1: 115-116.

Stinson, Charles, and Laguna Honda Hospital Bioethics Committee (1997). Interdisciplinary Care of Dying Persons: Information and Guideline Recommendations of the Laguna Honda Bioethics Committee: Revision: June 3, 1997.

Tinetti, M. (1986). Performance-oriented assessment of mobility problems in the elderly. Journal of the American Geriatrics Society. Vol. 34: 119-126.

Yesavage, J. et al. (1983). Development and Validation of a Geriatric Depression Screening Scale: A Preliminary Report. Journal of Psychiatric Research. Vol. 17: 37-49.

Caregivers and Professionals Partnership: A Hospital Based Program for Family Caregivers

Judy Dobrof, DSW
Bradley D. Zodikoff, MS
Helene Ebenstein, MSW
Debra Phillips, MS

SUMMARY. This article describes the Caregivers and Professionals Partnership (CAPP), a multi-faceted, interdisciplinary, replicable program model to strengthen and sustain the Mount Sinai Medical Center's responsiveness to the role and needs of family caregivers of adults. CAPP's three major programmatic components are: (1) the CAPP Caregiver Resource Center, (2) an Educational Program for caregivers and staff and (3) a Performance Improvement initiative. CAPP employs innovative outreach strategies to family caregivers of adults, including to

Judy Dobrof is Assistant Director of the Department of Social Work Services, Mount Sinai Medical Center. Bradley D. Zodikoff is Special Projects Coordinator, Caregivers and Professionals Partnership, Mount Sinai Medical Center. Helene Ebenstein is Coordinator at the CAPP Caregiver Resource Center, Mount Sinai Medical Center. Debra Phillips is a Social Worker at the CAPP Caregiver Resource Center, Mount Sinai Medical Center.

Address correspondence to: Judy Dobrof, DSW, Mount Sinai Medical Center, Department of Social Work Services, Box 1252, One Gustave L. Levy Place, New York, NY 10029 (E-mail: judy.dobrof@mountsinai.org).

[Haworth co-indexing entry note]: "Caregivers and Professionals Partnership: A Hospital Based Program for Family Caregivers." Dobrof, Judy et al. Co-published simultaneously in *Journal of Gerontological Social Work* (The Haworth Social Work Practice Press, an imprint of The Haworth Press, Inc.) Vol. 40, No. 1/2, 2002, pp. 23-40; and: *Older People and Their Caregivers Across the Spectrum of Care* (ed: Judith L. Howe) The Haworth Social Work Practice Press, an imprint of The Haworth Press, Inc., 2003, pp. 23-40. Single or multiple copies of this article are available for a fee from The Haworth Document Delivery Service [1-800-HAWORTH, 9:00 a.m. - 5:00 p.m. (EST). E-mail address: docdelivery@haworthpress.com].

monolingual Spanish-speaking caregivers. The CAPP "partnership" model, in which health care professionals and caregivers jointly participate in various dimensions of the program's development and implementation, is described in the context of building hospital based institutional support to meet family caregivers' complex needs. *[Article copies available for a fee from The Haworth Document Delivery Service: 1-800-HAWORTH. E-mail address: <docdelivery@haworthpress.com> Website: <http://www.HaworthPress.com>*

KEYWORDS. Family caregiving, caregivers of older adults, Spanish-speaking caregivers, caregiver needs assessment, caregiver service utilization, elderly, older adults, chronic illness, caregiver resource center, caregiver education, performance improvement

Family caregivers, the bedrock of the long term health care system in the United States, are increasingly expected to take on more responsibility for their relatives. This is especially true for caregivers of the elderly. As patients are discharged earlier from hospitals, need more intensive care and live longer with chronic illnesses, family members bear the enormous task of their care. Caring for a family member is associated with emotional and physical health problems, especially depression (Schulz, O'Brien, Bookwala, & Fleissner, 1995; Donaldson, Tarrier, & Burns, 1997), isolation and tension among family members (Stommel, Collins, & Given, 1994), and loss of income and job opportunities (Robinson, 1997; White-Means & Chollet, 1996). The estimated economic value of the care being provided by family caregivers is staggering. To replace this care with paid help would cost an estimated $196 billion annually (Arno, Levine, & Memmott, 1999). Since hospitals and other health care providers are shifting responsibility to unpaid family members to keep down the costs of healthcare, it is essential that family caregivers get the recognition and support they need from these providers and they be embraced as partners in the health care team (Given, Given, & Kozachik, 2001; Levine, 1998). In fact, no assessment is complete unless it takes into account the patient's family caregiver network, particularly for the geriatric patient. This article describes the efforts of Mount Sinai Medical Center, a large urban health care setting, to address the needs of family caregivers and to heighten health care professionals' awareness of the vital role that caregivers play in the health care arena.

The primary role of the family in healthcare is not new. Family members have always provided the bulk of home care and will continue to provide this unpaid care to their relatives. What has changed during the past twenty years is the intensity and duration of the care they are expected to give. With reduced hospital stays, patients, especially the elderly, are discharged with more skilled nursing needs, and require more help with personal care such as bathing and dressing (Corradetti & Hills, 1998; Shaugnessy & Kramer, 1990). Given that 71% of caregivers nationally report that they are caring for someone with a long-standing or chronic illness (National Alliance for Caregiving/AARP, 1997), providing support to families throughout the course of illness–from diagnosis to the bereavement phase–is essential. Models of support have only recently begun to emerge to address unmet needs of family caregivers of older adults (Mezey, Miller, & Linton-Nelson, 1999) as awareness grows about the hardships they face. Hospitals are an ideal place in which to develop model support programs, given their central role in caring for chronically and seriously-ill patients and their families (Levine, 1998). Hospital social work departments with expertise in psychosocial issues of older adults and their families, as well as in-program development and community-based services can take a leadership role in developing and implementing these model programs.

THE CAREGIVERS AND PROFESSIONALS PARTNERSHIP

The Caregivers and Professionals Partnership (CAPP) is a multi-faceted, interdisciplinary program to strengthen and sustain Mount Sinai Medical Center's responsiveness to the role and needs of family caregivers of adults (see Figure 1). CAPP's target populations are: (1) caregivers connected with Mount Sinai and its affiliates through the care of their adult family member, their own care, their residence in the local community, or their employment; and (2) Mount Sinai health care providers.

CAPP emerged out of a needs assessment conducted in 1998 of family caregivers of adults with a diverse range of medical and psychiatric diagnoses. With funding from the New York City-based United Hospital Fund, Mount Sinai's Department of Social Work Services conducted focus groups with family caregivers and health care professionals and a telephone survey of English and Spanish-speaking caregivers to assess caregivers' needs in the Mount Sinai community. When family caregivers were asked what services would be helpful to them, many came up with the same idea–"one stop shopping." Caregivers overwhelmingly wanted one place to call or visit which could provide assistance on any one caregiving issue. During focus groups and interviews caregivers described the frustrations of trying to get information on various programs, services and medical conditions, but not knowing where to turn for help. In addition, caregivers felt that they were not adequately trained for many caregiving tasks and that health care professionals often did not include them in decision-making nor recognize their valuable contribution to patients' care.

During the assessment phase, the following major needs were identified as relevant to a diverse range of caregivers of both hospitalized and community-dwelling patients: centralized information and support services; coordinated programs to advocate for caregivers; culturally-sensitive, bilingual services for Spanish-speaking caregivers; and education for health care providers. Therefore, CAPP developed as a comprehensive hospital-based program to raise awareness among health care professionals of the experiences and needs of family caregivers and to provide services to meet these needs.

CAPP has three major goals: (1) promote and sustain hospital-wide sensitivity and programmatic responses to caregivers' roles and needs; (2) provide centralized, culturally sensitive services to caregivers and their Mount Sinai health care providers; and (3) implement a model that can be replicated in other healthcare settings. CAPP has been implemented under the guidance of its Steering Committee composed of senior physicians, hospital staff, as well as caregivers.

CAPP includes three major programmatic components:

1. The *CAPP Caregiver Resource Center* which provides centralized, accessible information and support to caregivers of adult patients through telephone and walk-in assistance, a resource library, and website;
2. An *Education Program* for caregivers and staff to (a) enhance caregivers' ability to manage caring for family members and (b) provide staff training to improve hospital-wide practice with family caregivers; and
3. A *Performance Improvement* initiative to increase institutional responsiveness to caregiver issues.

CAPP CAREGIVER RESOURCE CENTER

Since September, 1999, the CAPP Caregiver Resource Center has provided information, referral, advocacy and support to family care-

FIGURE 1. Caregivers and Professionals Partnership

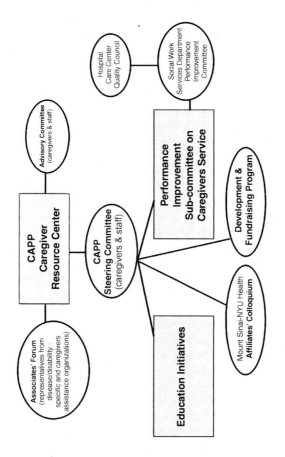

givers of adults. Located within the hospital setting, the Resource Center accepts referrals, phone calls, and visits from caregivers and professional staff. Services are available in English and Spanish. Caregivers contact the Resource Center seeking support and information, for example, about support groups, home care, adult day programs, assisted living, discharge issues, entitlements and many other related issues. The Center is staffed by two masters-level social workers, social work graduate interns and a cadre of volunteers, some of whom are family caregivers. An Advisory Committee composed of physicians, nurses, social workers, other Hospital staff as well as caregivers provides guidance to Resource Center staff.

The Resource Center is the Medical Center's central repository of information about resources, educational programs and supports for family caregivers within and outside of the institution. CAPP has built a comprehensive resource library of pamphlets, brochures, and books of interest to caregivers. Material from a wide range of hospital and agency-based programs, including community-based disease-specific organizations, is also available. Though information is an essential tool of the Resource Center, CAPP's programmatic philosophy emphasizes supportive, personalized, culturally sensitive and responsive services. From the initial contact, social workers focus on meeting the individualized needs of each caregiver who calls or visits. Some caregivers are calling for basic information, for example, about obtaining a list of home care agencies in their area. Others initially present with a simple request for information. However, upon further assessment, they are found to have complex needs that require interventions ranging from resource information to ongoing supportive counseling. Yet others present with complex needs from the start that require comprehensive psychosocial assessment and intervention.

For example, Ms. B. called the Caregiver Resource Center seeking information about home care and housing for her 80-year-old father who was diagnosed with Alzheimer's Disease. Although she focused only on these issues, there seemed to be other serious underlying problems involving relationships among family members and dealing with her father's very erratic behavior. Ms. B. brushed these topics aside. The social worker respected Ms. B's wishes and provided information on home care options, followed up and left the door open for further contacts. This allowed Ms. B. to contact the Resource Center when she was ready to talk about the tense relationships among her stepmother, other siblings and herself, her need to assume complete responsibility for her father and the stress of juggling caregiving, work, and marriage.

She obtained supportive counseling and is considering joining a support group.

An essential component of Resource Center services is a timely follow-up assessment to caregivers to provide ongoing support as their needs change and to insure that they have obtained the information or services they were seeking. Additionally, during this follow-up assessment, social workers obtain feedback regarding, for example, the helpfulness of agency services to which they were referred. Also important to caregivers is knowing that the Resource Center is there for them as they face other issues, some unexpected and others which naturally come up during the course of caregiving. By following-up routinely, the Resource Center maintains ongoing links with caregivers who are, for example, contemplating placing a family in a nursing home, locating a hospice program and, finally, needing bereavement counseling. Caregivers routinely express their appreciation for this on-going follow-up with statements such as "I can't believe someone cares about how *I* am doing."

The Resource Center's knowledge base and community roots are strengthened by its links to a group of disease-specific and caregiver assistance organizations (e.g., Alzheimers' Association and Well Spouse Foundation) that are part of the CAPP Caregiver Resource Center Associates Forum. The Associates Forum meets periodically, providing an efficient way to keep current on various agencies' caregiver programs. The Forum is also used to publicize Resource Center services and facilitate caregiver referrals to Forum members.

Collecting data on each caregiver contact has allowed CAPP to accurately monitor Resource Center usage, identify trends in caregivers' presenting issues, document gaps in services identified by family caregivers, and monitor outcomes of Resource Center referrals and other services for performance improvement purposes. This information is presented to the CAPP Steering and Advisory Committees that can advocate for Hospital-wide and legislative responsiveness to caregivers' needs. To track each caregiver contact, CAPP created a data record to identify salient information about each Resource Center contact. Based on data collected since September 1999, caregivers who have contacted the Resource Center have been mostly female, ranging in age from 18-93, and representing many family relationships including adult children, spouses, grandchildren and friends. Among those caregivers who reported their ages, 60% are over age 60. For care recipients whose ages were reported, 70% of care recipients are 60 years old or older; of those, 50% are over 80 years old. While the Resource Center fields questions from all adult age groups, the majority of caregivers and especially care recipients clearly comprise an older population. Diagnoses of care recipients vary and include: dementia, cardiac disease, depression, cancer, Parkinson's disease, stroke, diabetes and fractures. Often, care recipients have multiple impairments. This data continues to support the need for a centralized Resource Center, able to address a wide range of caregiver types and issues.

The data collection process enables CAPP to accumulate information from caregivers about specific problems, service gaps and barriers. For example, many caregivers express anxiety due to inadequate information about the care recipient's medical condition/prognosis and specific care needed. Many caregivers worry about the cost of long-term care and they often take on more caregiving responsibilities than they can handle in an effort to make savings last. There also appears to be a lack of support groups specifically for caregivers (many groups combine patients and caregivers) which are conveniently located and deal with general caregiver issues. Questions about affordable housing for seniors (e.g., assisted living facilities, enriched housing) highlight the lack of options in the New York area for care recipients who can no longer remain in their homes. When caregivers whose relatives recently died seek bereavement counseling services, these services are often difficult to locate. The need for bereavement services following the transition from the caregiving role represents a major service gap. Finally, the barriers facing caregivers who do not speak English represent a serious problem. The lack of services such as support groups, day programs and educational workshops for Spanish-speaking caregivers and others who do not speak English is another critical service gap.

EDUCATIONAL INITIATIVES

CAPP Caregiver Institute

Once the Caregiver Resource Center was in place, CAPP obtained additional UHF funding to create the CAPP Caregiver Institute as a new educational program for family caregivers. The purpose of the Caregiver Institute is to provide family caregivers with knowledge, skills, and support to manage their caregiving responsibilities. Through a "partnership model," family caregivers with a particular expertise are paired with health care professionals to teach each workshop. Caregiver experts gain opportunities to share their knowledge with other caregivers who participate in Institute workshops. Workshops focus on specific topics such as home care, financial and legal concerns, entitlements and benefits, technical training on "hands on" care of the patient and caregiver stress and coping.

CAPP developed the Institute based on caregivers' frequent requests for more information and formalized training to assist in managing caregiving tasks. Caregivers often express the need for education about a range of issues from better understanding their family member's illness to knowing how to provide hands-on care. Many caregivers talk about how poorly prepared they feel for handling the crises and challenges of caregiving, both in the hospital and at home, and how education and information may have helped with much of the anxiety many caregivers experienced in taking on new and vital responsibilities for which they had little or no training. For many caregivers, workshops are not only educational, but also help them to manage their caregiving tasks.

Many experienced "long-term" caregivers gain enormous expertise in the caregiving role over time. The sharing of information, resources, challenges, rewards, and coping strategies caregiver-to-caregiver is an effective model of education and support even within a single session format. Therefore, the Caregiver Institute's use of caregiver-volunteer "experts" to communicate specific skills, knowledge, information, and support *to other caregivers* provides institutional recognition of caregivers' special skills and strengths while simultaneously promoting an educational model based on reciprocal, mutual support. Pairing caregiver-volunteers with health care professionals as Caregiver Institute Faculty is the cornerstone of the Caregiver Institute's educational model.

In fact, health-care professionals' and caregivers' experiences served to complement one another effectively in many workshops. For example, in a workshop on financial concerns, a benefits and entitlements expert from the hospital presented a sophisticated method for organizing and managing a patient's financial and legal documents (e.g., bank accounts, living will, health care proxy). The experienced caregiver on the panel also detailed her own method for organizing her mother's financial affairs. In the course of the presentation, the caregiver shared how she coped with some of the emotional issues and challenges associated with assuming the role of "financial manager" and "healthcare proxy" to her ailing mother, who due to Alzheimer's disease, was no longer able to manage financial and healthcare decisions for herself. The caregiver explained how she had to confront her own feelings of discomfort, sadness and loss before she could begin to intervene effectively in the financial affairs of her mother who had always maintained independence and complete privacy in this dimension of her life. Workshop attendees responded positively to the different perspectives of the healthcare professional and caregiver on the panel, as evidenced by attendee participation and discussion as well as in the written evaluations following each workshop.

Medical Student Practice Enhancement

Through a grant from the Mount Sinai School of Medicine, a newly designed curriculum on family caregivers was implemented to enhance medical students' understanding of the experiences and needs of family caregivers. Using lectures, a panel discussion by family caregivers, including a medical student who had cared for her terminally-ill mother, videotapes of family caregiver focus groups, and small group discussions, students gain a greater awareness of the challenges that family caregivers face. Role plays of physician/family caregiver interactions were also developed as a method of improving students' skills in working with caregivers. Course directors have requested that the curriculum become a permanent part of a newly designed course for first-and second-year medical students called, "The Art and Science of Medicine."

THE DEPARTMENT OF SOCIAL WORK SERVICE'S PERFORMANCE IMPROVEMENT COMMITTEE ON CAREGIVER SERVICES

In a time of shrinking resources and enormous time constraints, it was critical to design a program that capitalized on existing, common mechanisms for improving care. Every healthcare institution is mandated, both by the Joint Commission on Accreditation of Healthcare Organizations (JCAHO) and regulatory agencies, to have a performance improvement structure, which reports to the CEO and Board of Trustees. That structure, and the standards by which institutions are evaluated, have an enormous influence on institutional priorities and resource allocation.

Therefore, the Department of Social Work Services created a Committee on Caregiver Services as part of its performance improvement program. The committee includes social worker representation from all areas of the Hospital and focuses on enhancing social work practice with family caregivers of adults. The Committee reports regularly to the

Department of Social Work Services Performance Improvement Committee which forwards quarterly reports to the Hospital Care Center Quality Council. The Council sends regular reports to the Patient Care Committee of the Medical Center's Board of Trustees. This structure serves as a model for other disciplines concerned with practice enhancement with family caregivers. The mandated formal reporting structure has served as an additional venue in which to heighten institutional awareness of family caregiver issues.

The Performance Improvement Committee has systematically examined social workers' practice with family caregivers by developing a Caregiver Quality Indicator data collection tool for use in a comprehensive representative chart review. Committee members were especially interested in whether chart documentation reflected caregivers' involvement in decision making and whether caregivers were provided with information, education, and support, standards that have been developed by the United Hospital Fund to guide relationships between healthcare professionals and families (United Hospital Fund, 1998). This is especially critical for caregivers of older adults who many times face the responsibility of providing the major portion of care at home.

Through chart review and discussion with social workers throughout the Medical Center, Committee members found: (1) social workers across all areas frequently include family caregivers in decision-making regarding the patient's plan of care, but less frequently focus on how caregivers are coping with assuming and managing their caregiving responsibilities; (2) lack of time and private space in which to speak with families about confidential matters are major obstacles to work with caregivers. However, social workers also recognized that, due to the lack of time, documentation does not always capture fully social workers' practice with families. In other words, many times they are interacting extensively with families, but do not always document their work. Working within an interdisciplinary team that focuses on patients *and* families facilitate their ability to focus on families.

From these findings, Committee members are developing recommendations to standardize psychosocial assessment forms to include family resource needs *and* coping capacities as major categories for attention by social workers. Other social workers have included enhanced work with families as a goal in their yearly performance appraisal.

OUTREACH TO FAMILY CAREGIVERS

The CAPP program has marketed services to family caregivers in numerous ways, as reaching family caregivers in need has been a consistently challenging and labor-intensive task. CAPP has employed a two-pronged strategy to reach out to family caregivers: (1) by soliciting referrals from health care and social service professionals who interact with family caregivers in their clinical practice and (2) by targeting family caregivers directly. CAPP has marketed its services to professionals and family caregivers both within the Mount Sinai health care system as well as in the community at large.

Though the CAPP program has been successful reaching a large number of family caregivers, our experience confirms that family caregivers are in fact very difficult to reach. Marketing and outreach involve constant, continuous, time-consuming efforts. One of our major programmatic concerns is distinguishing between those family caregivers who have identified the need for service and taken "the next step" by actively contacting the Resource Center and the much larger "hidden" population of family caregivers who, for a variety of reasons, do not actively seek any type of assistance. Some caregivers prefer no outside help. However, others would take advantage of available resources but are unaware of the array of services and programs available to assist them.

One of the major barriers in reaching caregivers is the problem of "self-identification" or "self-definition" (Montgomery & Kosloski, 2001). Since many caregivers do not identify themselves as "caregivers," they do not realize there are services available to assist them. Therefore, helping people to see themselves as caregivers, while also helping them to locate supportive services, has been a critical focus of CAPP's ongoing outreach work.

Fundamental to these outreach efforts is the need to clearly define the term "caregiver." CAPP defines "caregiver" broadly to include, for example, people who are just beginning to worry about an aging parent or spouse as well as those who have been performing hands-on care for years. Family members often respond that they are not caregivers because, for example, they do not bathe or toilet a relative. Others explain that they are not the "primary" caregiver, not paid, don't live close by or offer a host of other reasons why they do not see themselves as caregivers despite their often extensive involvement with family members. CAPP staff members continually educate caregivers about the range of caregiving roles and always explain the term in written material, workshops, and in caregiver contacts.

The Discharge Follow-Up Program is another strategy for reaching out to caregivers who may not ask for assistance. Under this program, CAPP Resource Center staff contact: (1) those referred by Mount Sinai or community staff because they were considered "at risk" as they were having difficulty coping and/or had need for resources such as home care or a respite program and (2) those patients discharged from Mount Sinai to sub-acute facilities (e.g., rehabilitation centers). This group was particularly targeted for outreach because the transition from hospital to home can be so difficult for the caregiver as well as the patient. Response to this program has been very positive. Many of the caregivers contacted have identified needs for which they had not sought help previously. The Discharge Follow-up Program provides an example of an outreach strategy whereby the Resource Center actively seeks contact with potentially high-risk caregivers, rather than just "waiting" for high-risk caregivers to call.

Highlighting the role of family caregivers to hospital staff is another way of enhancing identification of caregivers. CAPP program staff have worked intensively within the hospital to emphasize the importance of family caregivers. Unit meetings, grand rounds, newsletter articles all help remind staff about family caregivers and the CAPP program. Recognizing that many hospital employees are also family caregivers and encouraging them to use CAPP services has also been effective.

REACHING SPANISH-SPEAKING CAREGIVERS

Since Mount Sinai Hospital is located in East Harlem, a predominantly Spanish-speaking community in New York City, the CAPP Program has specifically focused on addressing the needs of Latino caregivers. An additional grant from the James N. Jarvie Commonweal Service funded a Spanish-speaking bicultural social worker to provide direct services and to heighten awareness of Spanish-speaking family caregivers' special concerns. In focus groups and a telephone survey as well as in ongoing Resource Center contacts, Spanish-speaking caregivers have reported multiple obstacles in accessing services. These obstacles include, for example, the lack of Spanish-speaking health care professionals in hospitals and community programs and the absence of culturally-sensitive services to meet their needs.

The language barrier is the most common obstacle monolingual Spanish-speaking caregivers face in seeking community services (Delgado & Tennstedt, 1997; Tennstedt, Chang, & Delgado, 1998) and interacting with health and social service professionals. This population of caregivers face special challenges due to the paucity of linguistically and culturally-appropriate services. For example, the CAPP Caregiver Resource Center bilingual social worker provides resource information, referral, and support through individual counseling. Many caregivers contact the Caregiver Resource Center requesting assistance in locating support groups and educational programs in Spanish. As for many caregivers, these kinds of programs are essential in helping them manage their caregiving responsibilities. However, very few programs exist in New York City specifically for Spanish-speaking caregivers. Therefore, in response to this need, CAPP developed a caregiver support group and educational workshops led in Spanish. Additionally, CAPP's Associates Forum of disease-specific and caregiver assistance organizations has focused on strategies to increase programming for this population.

The issue of caregiver self-identification, as with other caregivers, also impedes many Latino caregivers' use of available services. Caring for an ill relative is engrained in Latino cultures, incorporating the notion of "respeto" (respect) towards parents and elders (Calderón and Tennstedt, 1998, Sánchez-Ayéndez, 1998). Elder Spanish-speaking caregivers are particularly reluctant to self-identify as they view caring for a family member as natural and unquestioned (Delgado & Tennstedt, 1997).

Therefore, CAPP has implemented a multi-faceted community outreach strategy targeting monolingual Spanish-speaking caregivers at Mount Sinai and in the community. One important dimension of outreach work has focused on alerting Mount Sinai health care providers to the availability of Spanish-language caregiver services for their patients' families. Another focus is creating and building awareness in the community surrounding Mount Sinai about Mount Sinai Caregiver Resource Center services in Spanish. Developing ongoing relationships with key contacts in the community has been a critical outreach strategy. Examples include clergy, elected officials, and social service providers. In addition, CAPP developed and disseminated educational materials in both English and Spanish, since so little caregiver educational material has been written in Spanish.

In summary, interventions with Spanish-speaking caregivers, all of which emphasize educational tasks, include: (1) formally educating individuals about the definition and identity of "caregiver" so that they begin to make the connection between the common problems they are experiencing *as caregivers* and the fact that there are services available to address some of these common problems, (2) creating awareness about the specific programs and services available to assist Spanish-speaking caregivers, and (3) facilitating caregivers' access to these services through brief counseling as well as through intensive advocacy.

DISCUSSION

CAPP has been highly successful as a multi-faceted approach to raising institutional awareness of the experiences of family caregivers and developing programmatic responses to their unmet needs. One of CAPP's greatest strengths is its focus on service provision to family caregivers of adults *across all disease categories* and *across the entire spectrum of care*. As a hospital-based caregiver initiative, CAPP recognized from its inception that the lack of centralized information and support services remains a key obstacle to meeting caregivers' multiple needs within the health care system. Caregivers seek a wide variety of resources and often do not know where to turn for assistance either within or outside the health care system. The CAPP Caregiver Resource Center has strategically marketed itself as a *comprehensive, centralized* repository of information that will provide *all* family caregivers of adults in the health care system with specifically-tailored information, referral, advocacy and counseling services. By marketing itself as a unique, comprehensive *hospital-wide* program, rather than as a specific program of any one department or disease-specific area, CAPP offers family caregivers a simple, easy to identify, direct "point-of-entry" into the maze of support services available within the institution and in the community at large. Being a hospital-wide program also resulted in critical support from multiple hospital departments and from staff in key areas of the hospital.

Another strength of the CAPP program is its systems-oriented, multi-faceted focus on resource center services, educational programs, and hospital-based performance improvement initiatives. While direct service provision and education for family caregivers are the core foci of the CAPP program, equally important, both substantively and philosophically, is CAPP's focus on building staff awareness about family caregiver issues and working towards creating a professional "culture-shift" to enhance institutional responsiveness to family caregivers' needs. Involving family caregivers, physicians and hospital staff in all aspects of the program has strengthened the program, giving it increased credibility, and led to a gradual heightened awareness of the experiences and needs of family caregivers. This culture shift is apparent in the number of staff who refer family members with whom they are working as well as use the resource center for assistance with their own caregiving needs. The program has been recognized by Mount Sinai as exemplary as demonstrated for example by the ongoing involvement and commitment of its Steering Committee. In 2000, as part of the JCAHO survey process, it was showcased as a "best practice" among Mount Sinai programs.

Caregiver participation in particular is a cornerstone of CAPP's "partnership" model and has added a tangible dimension of vitality, relevance, and legitimacy to the program. As one caregiver said during the planning phase, "Treat us like partners, not pests!" CAPP was designed to put this statement into action by, for example, including caregivers on its Steering Committee, as faculty members of its Caregiver Institute, and as volunteers in its Resource Center. At a time when customer satisfaction has become critical to quality health care, caregiver input has contributed to CAPP's success as a program to meet caregivers' needs. For example, family caregivers have contributed to the development of the Resource Center pamphlet to ensure its clarity. They have also contributed to the development of programs that are relevant and user-friendly.

CAPP has provided essential information, support, and advocacy services to family caregivers which, in turn, is critical to the fiscal health of the Hospital. The hospital has drawn on family caregivers' assistance to discharge patients quickly and prevent further hospitalizations and emergency department visits. Many patients are maintained at home only through the involvement of family caregivers who provide direct assistance and/or care coordination. Considering that it has been found that in the year following a hospitalization the level of care that caregivers provide dramatically increases (Levine, 2000), hospital based programs such as CAPP are integral to supporting family caregivers.

REFERENCES

Arno, P.S., Levine, C., & Memmott, M.M. (1999). The economic value of informal caregiving. *Health Affairs, 18* (2), 182-188.

Calderón, V., & Tennstedt, S. (1998). Ethnic differences in the expression of caregiver burden: Results of a qualitative study. *Journal of Gerontological Social Work, 30* (1/2), 159-178.

Corradetti, E.V., & Hills, G.A. (1998). Assessing and supporting caregivers of the elderly. *Topics in Geriatric Rehabilitation, 14*(1), 12-35.

Cummings, S.M. (1996). Spousal caregivers of early stage Alzheimer's patients: A psychoeducational support group model. *Journal of Gerontological Social Work, 26* (3/4), 83-98.

Delgado, M., & Tennstedt, S. (1997). Making the case for culturally appropriate community services: Puerto Rican elders and their caregivers. *Health and Social Work, 22* (4), 246-255.

Donaldson, C., Tarrier, N., & Burns, A., (1997). The impact of the symptoms of dementia on caregivers. *British Journal of Psychiatry, 170,* 62-8.

Esmail, R., Brazil, K., & Lam, M., (2000). Short report. Compliance with recommendations in a geriatric outreach assessment service. *Age and Ageing, 29,* 353-356.

Feder, J., Komisar, H.L., & Niefeld, M. (2000). Long-term care in the United States: An overview. *Health Affairs, 19* (3), 40-56.

Fredman, L., & Daly, M.P. (1998). Enhancing practitioner ability to recognize and treat caregiver physical and mental consequences. *Topics in Geriatric Rehabilitation, 14* (1), 36-44.

Given, B.A., Given, C.W., & Kozachik, S. (2001). Family support in advanced cancer. *CA A Cancer Journal for Clinicians, 51* (4), 213-231.

Gormley, N. (2000). The role of dementia training programmes in reducing care-giver burden. *Psychiatric Bulletin, 24,* 41-42.

Hills, G.A. (1998). Caregivers of the elderly: Hidden patients and health team members. *Topics in Geriatric Rehabilitation, 14* (1), 1-11.

Houts, P.S., Nezu, A.M., Nezu, C.M., & Bucher, J.A. (1996). The prepared family caregiver: A problem-solving approach to family caregiver education. *Patient Education and Counseling, 27,* 63-73.

Huston, P.G. (1990). Family care of the elderly and caregiver stress. *American Family Physician, 42,* 671-676.

Levine, C. (1998). *Rough crossings: Family caregivers' odysseys through the health care system.* New York: United Hospital Fund of New York.

Levine, C., Kuerbis, A., Gould, D., Navie-Waliser, M., Hollander Feldman, P., & Donelan, K. (2000). *A survey of family caregivers in New York City: Findings and implications for the health care system.* United Hospital Fund & Visiting Nurse Service of New York.

Liu, K., Manton, K. G., & Aragon, C. (2000). Changes in home care use by disabled elderly persons: 1982-1994. *Journal of Gerontology: Social Sciences, 55B* (4), S245-253.

Mezey, M., Miller, L.L., & Linton-Nelson, L. (1999). Caring for caregivers of frail elders at the end of life. *Generations, 23* (1), 44-51.

Montgomery, R., & Kosloski, K. (2001). Change, continuity and diversity among caregivers. In *The National Family Caregiver Support Program: From enactment to action: U.S. Administration on Aging Conference: Selected issue briefs.* (September, 2001).Washington, DC.

National Alliance for Caregiving & AARP. (1997*). Family Caregiving in the U.S.: Findings from a national survey.* Washington, D.C.: Author.

Navaie-Waliser, M. (2001). The experiences and challenges of informal caregivers: Common themes, and differences among Whites, Blacks, and Hispanics. *The Gerontologist, 41* (6), 733-740.

Ostwald, S.K., Hepburn, K.W., Caron,W., Burns, T., & Mantell R. (1999) Reducing caregiver burden: A randomized psychoeducational intervention for caregivers of persons with dementia. *The Gerontologist, 39,* 299-309.

Robinson, K.M. (1997). The family's role in long-term care. *Journal of Gerontological Nursing, 23* (9), 7-11.

Sánchez-Ayéndez, M. (1998). Middle-aged Puerto Rican women as primary caregivers to the elderly: A qualitative analysis of everyday dynamics. *Journal of Gerontological Social Work, 30* (1/2): 75-97.

Schulz, R., O'Brien, A.T., Bookwala, J., & Fleissner, K. (1995) Psychiatric and physical morbidity effects of dementia caregiving: Prevalence, correlates, and causes. *The Gerontologist, 35,* 771-791.

Shaugnessy, P.W. & Kramer, R.M. (1990). The increased needs of patients in nursing home and patients receiving home health care. *New England Journal of Medicine, 322:* 21-27.

Stommel, M., Collins, C.E., & Given, C.W. (1994). The costs of family contributions to the care of persons with dementia. *The Gerontologist, 34*(2), 199-205.

Tennstedt, S., Chang, B-H., & Delgado, M. (1998) Patterns of long-term care: A comparison of Puerto Rican, African-American, and Non-Latino White elders. *Journal of Gerontological Social Work, 30* (1/2) : 179-199.

Toseland, R.W., & McCallion, P. (1997). Trends in caregiving intervention research. *Social Work Research, 21*(3), 154-164.

Weuve, J.L., Boult, C., & Morishita, L. (2000). The effects of outpatient geriatric evaluation and management on caregiver burden. *The Gerontologist, 40*(4) 429-436.

White-Means, S., & Chollet, D. (1996). Opportunity wages and workforce adjustments: Understanding the cost of in-home elder care. *Journal of Gerontology: Social Sciences, 51B,* S82-S90.

Older Adults with HIV Disease: Challenges for Integrated Assessment

Charles A. Emlet, PhD, MSW
Susan Scott Gusz, PHN
Jodi Dumont, MSW

SUMMARY. Persons age 50 and over have consistently accounted for 10-15% of all cases of AIDS in the United States reported to the Centers for Disease Control and Prevention. With increased longevity due to antiretroviral medications, we can expect to see increasing numbers of older adults living with HIV and AIDS in the coming years. This newly emerging vulnerable population requires an understanding and sound clinical response that incorporates the needs of both older adults in general and persons living with HIV/AIDS. If older adults with HIV/AIDS are to receive sound assessments from professional social workers, an integration of knowledge from these two, up to now, different arenas of practice will need to occur.

Charles A. Emlet is Assistant Professor of Social Work at the University of Washington, Tacoma and a Hartford Geriatric Social Work Faculty Scholar. Susan Scott Gusz is Public Health Nurse and Nurse Case Manager, AIDS Case Management Program, Older and Disabled Adult Unit, Solano County Health and Social Services, Fairfield, CA. Jodi Dumont is Case Manager, Pierce County AIDS Foundation, Tacoma, WA.

Address correspondence to: Dr. Emlet at 1900 Commerce Street, Campus Box 358425, Tacoma, WA 98402 (E-mail: caemlet@u.washington.edu).

[Haworth co-indexing entry note]: "Older Adults with HIV Disease: Challenges for Integrated Assessment." Emlet, Charles A., Susan Scott Gusz, and Jodi Dumont. Co-published simultaneously in *Journal of Gerontological Social Work* (The Haworth Social Work Practice Press, an imprint of The Haworth Press, Inc.) Vol. 40, No. 1/2, 2002, pp. 41-62; and: *Older People and Their Caregivers Across the Spectrum of Care* (ed: Judith L. Howe) The Haworth Social Work Practice Press, an imprint of The Haworth Press, Inc., 2003, pp. 41-62. Single or multiple copies of this article are available for a fee from The Haworth Document Delivery Service [1-800-HAWORTH, 9:00 a.m. - 5:00 p.m. (EST). E-mail address: docdelivery@haworthpress.com].

http://www.haworthpress.com/store/product.asp?sku=J083
10.1300/J083v40n01_04

KEYWORDS. Aging, older adults, older persons, HIV/AIDS, HIV disease, geriatric assessment, vulnerable populations, at-risk populations, interdisciplinary, social work

Older adults often defined in HIV research as those age 50 years and over, are increasingly recognized as being at-risk for HIV disease. HIV/AIDS has traditionally been seen as a disease of younger persons. Thus, older adults with HIV/AIDS have been called a "hidden population" (Emlet, 1997) and the "invisible ten percent" (Genke, 2000) referring to the fact that approximately 10% of AIDS cases in the United States diagnosed in persons age 50 and over. No matter the setting or primary client population, social work practitioners will likely meet and work with older persons and persons with HIV/AIDS. Since both aging and HIV disease are ubiquitous in social work practice, social workers will increasingly need to be prepared to provide assessment and other social work services to older persons who are infected with and affected by HIV disease (Emlet & Poindexter, 2002).

The purpose of this paper is twofold. First, the authors will present the reader with important demographic and epidemiological trends related to older adults and HIV/AIDS, providing social workers in general, and gerontological social workers specifically, with updated information and knowledge about this emerging vulnerable population. Second, we will provide an overview of the important elements essential to effective assessment of older adults as well as persons living with HIV/AIDS. We will then combine those elements and present a model for the assessment of older adults living with HIV/AIDS.

HIV/AIDS IN OLDER PERSONS: AN OVERVIEW

Epidemiology

As of June 2001, 793,026 cases of AIDS were reported in the United States. Of those, 86,875 or 11 percent were diagnosed in people age 50 or older (CDC, 2002). This figure does not include those diagnosed with AIDS at a younger age who have "aged in" with the disease nor does it include people age 50 or older who have been diagnosed HIV+, but have not yet progressed to AIDS. According to Wooten-Bielski (1999) the figure of 11 percent may under-represent actual number of cases because AIDS goes undiagnosed in older people to a larger degree than in their younger counterparts. Because of the lack of accurate diagnosis, it is possible that many infected older adults die without having been diagnosed (Szirony, 1999). As medical treatments extend life expectancy for those with HIV and as the population of older adults increases, the number of HIV/AIDS cases among older adults are expected to increase (Genke, 2000, Wooten-Bielski, 1999; Poindexter & Linsk, 2000).

As shown in Table 1, the reported modes of transmission among people aged 50 and older are similar to those aged 13 to 49, with people aged 50+ slightly more likely to report unknown or unreported risk, heterosexual contact, and blood products (CDC, 1998; Inungu, Mokotoff & Kent, 2001). While initially, reports of infection through tainted blood products among older adults were significantly higher, the implementation of more stringent donor guidelines and routine screening of blood donations in 1985 resulted in marked decrease in the number of cases reported with this risk factor (CDC, 1998). The numbers of AIDS cases associated with other modes of exposure, however, have increased in older adults (CDC, 1998). While the overall proportion of cases of AIDS in those 50 and older has remained fairly constant since the mid-1980s, the actual number of cases has risen dramatically (Zelenetz & Epstein, 1998).

With regard to gender, older women, particularly older women of color, continue to be at risk for HIV (Emlet, Tangenberg, & Siverson,

TABLE 1. AIDS cases in the US, by age group and exposure category in 1996.

HIV exposure category	> 50 years n = 7,459	13-49 years n = 61,014
Men who have sex with men (MSM)	35.9%	40.4%
Injection drug use (IDU)	19.2%	25.6%
MSM and IDU	2.2%	4.6%
Heterosexual contact	14.5%	12.7%
Blood products	2.4%	1.1%
No risk reported	25.8%	15.6%

Source: Centers For Disease Control and Prevention, MMWR, 1998, 47(2), 21-26.

2002). As shown in Table 2, the proportion of AIDS cases in African American women, age 50 and older is more than double that of white women. Latina women, representing a smaller population than either White or African American women are diagnosed at similar numbers to Whites in the 50-54 and 55-59 age ranges. Regarding ethnicity, of the total number of cases in people age 50 or older, 45% are White, 38% are Black, 16% are Hispanic, 1% is Asian/Pacific Islander, and less than .5% are American Indian/Alaska Native (CDC, 2002).

Risk Factors for Older Adults

Like all people, older adults are at-risk for contracting HIV/AIDS when there is a history of unprotected sex with male or female partners (including vaginal, oral, and anal sex); blood transfusions between 1977 and 1985; sexual activity with prostitutes, intravenous drug use, and

TABLE 2. AIDS cases by sex, age at diagnosis, and ethnicity in people ages 50 and over as of June 2001, United States.

Male age at diagnosis (years)	White, not Hispanic	Black, not Hispanic	Hispanic	Asian/ Pacific Islander	American Indian/ Alaska Native	Total[1]
	n (%)	n (%)	n (%)	n (%)	n (%)	n (%)
50-54	17,047 (48)	12,265 (48)	5,618 (48)	288 (48)	59 (46)	35,312 (48)
55-59	9,123 (26)	6,689 (26)	3,067 (26)	168 (28)	34 (27)	19,122 (26)
60-64	5,023 (14)	3,650 (14)	1,711 (15)	74 (12)	18 (14)	10,483 (14)
65 or older	4,130 (12)	3,090 (12)	1,388 (11)	73 (12)	16 (13)	8,707 (12)
Male subtotal	35,323 (100)	25,694 (100)	11,784 (100)	603 (100)	127 (100)	73,624 (100)
Female age at diagnosis (years)						
50-54	1,233 (36)	3,199 (46)	1,173 (45)	31 (27)	21 (45)	5,660 (43)
55-59	783 (22)	1,755 (25)	719 (28)	27 (24)	16 (35)	3,301 (25)
60-64	497 (14)	1,023 (15)	378 (14)	28 (25)	5 (11)	1,932 (14)
65 or older	973 (28)	1,021 (14)	330 (13)	27 (24)	4 (9)	2,358 (18)
Female subtotal	3,486 (100)	6,998 (100)	2,600 (100)	113 (100)	46 (100)	13,251 (100)
Total	38,809 (45)	32,692 (38)	14,384 (16)	716 (1)	173 (<. 5)	86,875

Source: Centers For Disease Control and Prevention, HIV/AIDS Surveillance Report, 2002.
[1]Includes 93 males and 8 females whose race/ethnicity is unknown.

sexual activity with a partner who is at risk for infection (Wooten-Bielski, 1999). Older adults are at increased risk because the efficiency of the immune system of older adults has been reduced through age related decline (Szirony, 1999). Older women, who are no longer concerned about pregnancy, may not see a need for condom use. However, women who are post menopausal are actually at greater risk because their estrogen loss results in thinning of the vaginal mucosa, leaving them more susceptible to tears of the vaginal walls during sexual activity (Linsk, 2000; Szirony, 1999; Zelenetz & Epstein, 1998). Recently such risks have been "compounded by the surge in Viagra use among older men, who often receive the drug without receiving HIV prevention messages" (AIDS Action Council, 2001, p. 3). Despite their significant representation in persons diagnosed with HIV/AIDS, there is an assumption among medical practitioners and older adults that they are not at risk for HIV infection. Health care providers may feel uncomfortable discussing sexual issues with their older patients (Wooten-Bielski, 1999), or erroneously assume older individuals are not sexually active. Thus, important questions related to sexual activity and history may be omitted from medical assessments (Johnson, Haight, Faan, & Benedict, 1998). Similarly, older adults may be reluctant to disclose behaviors they view as being socially unacceptable. This may be especially true of older gay or bisexual men who have felt a need to hide their sexual identity throughout their lives in order to protect themselves from stigma and discrimination (Szirony, 1999; Wooten-Bielski, 1999). Such ageist attitudes reinforce these false perceptions resulting in older people having limited knowledge of HIV and prevention practices (Linsk, 2000).

Medical Concerns

The weakened immune system in older adults that leads to greater susceptibility of HIV infection may result in a more rapid progression of the disease (Wooten-Bielski, 1999). Numerous studies have found shorter survival times among older persons (Ferro and Salit, 1992; Inungu, Mokotoff, & Kent, 2001) and higher rates of mortality (CDC, 1998; Emlet & Farkas, 2002). Early diagnosis, however, provides elders with the best chance for effective treatment and a positive prognosis. Unfortunately, physicians continue to have low clinical suspicion for HIV in the elderly (Zelenetz & Epstein, 1998). This, combined with the fact that many AIDS related symptoms imitate medical problems that are common in older adults may lead to delayed or misdiagnosis and thus, delayed treatment (Johnson, Haight, Faan, & Benedict, 1998).

Psychosocial Considerations

Older adults with HIV/AIDS experience many of the same psychosocial issues as their younger counterparts, such as feeling stigmatized, marginalized and afraid (Linsk, 2000). They may fear disclosing their diagnosis, and experience strained relationships with family and friends (Zelenetz & Epstein, 1998). They may experience lack of support from the community, dwindling financial resources, and diminished quality of life (Szirony, 1999).

Older people with HIV/AIDS experience difficulties specific to their age group (Johnson, Haight, Faan, & Benedict, 1998) and may have lost multiple partner(s) and friends resulting in diminished social support. They may experience complicated bereavement, and feelings of "survivor guilt" (Genke, 2000, p. 203). Older adults can be caught between aging and HIV services, where their HIV issues may not be addressed by aging programs, while AIDS support services are typically geared to a younger population (Genke, 2000). In addition to facing discrimination based on HIV status, sex, and/or sexual identity, older adults must struggle with the effects of an ageist society. As Fowler (1999) describes, "in a society that does not respect or value the aging population, older HIV infected people may confront social and professional bias regarding allocation of health care services and resources available to the AIDS community" (p. 4). Research suggests older adults (with HIV) experience higher levels of depression than their younger HIV+ counterparts (Heckman, Kochman, Sikkema, & Kalichman, 1999). While this does not mean that HIV infected older people are incapable of adjusting to their HIV disease, it does mean that further research is warranted and that services must be available to support the unique needs of older HIV+ adults (Heckman, Heckman, Kochman, Sikkema, Suhr, & Goodkin, 2002).

Clearly, older adults face additional and different challenges regarding HIV/AIDS than their younger counterparts. As a result, it is essential that practitioners incorporate the important elements of a geriatric assessment with the elements of an HIV assessment. Such integration will result in a more thorough understanding of the needs of HIV+ older adults.

THE ASSESSMENT PROCESS

Gerontological social workers are familiar with the concept of assessment. Rubenstein (1987) defines geriatric assessment as a multidimensional, usually interdisciplinary process designed to quantify the elderly individual's medical, psychosocial, and functional capabilities.) Assessment "plays a central role in the evolution of the geriatric care system with regard to the integration of community programs and medical services for older persons with complex problems" (Urdangarin, 2000, p. 383). Such problems are exacerbated when adding the spectrum of issues associated with HIV disease to the already complicated aging process.

Geron (1997) provides us with several important characteristics to consider when conducting assessments. He suggests that assessments should: (1) *Be comprehensive in scope.* An adequate information base must include the client's problems, needs, resources and strengths; (2) *Be functional in design.* The assessment should support clinical decision making; (3) *Incorporate standardized measures.* Measures that have been tested for sound psychometric properties should be used; (4) *Balance psychometric precision with practicality.* The accuracy of what instruments measure (validity and reliability) must be balanced with the burden the assessment places on clients and families; (5) *Incorporate objective and multiple sources of information.* Assessments should rely on items that can be observed as well as demonstrated by the older adult. With client permission, information from other sources should be incorporated into the process; (6) *Assessments should be standardized across users.* Using a uniform assessment protocol facilitates interventions and decision making; (7) *Assessments should be easy to read and administer.* The use of technical language should be avoided when communicating with clients; (8) *Assessments should be culturally sensitive.* Assessors need to understand how cultural differences may affect healthcare access and utilization as well as assessor bias.

Geriatric Assessment

In conducting assessments with older adults, various areas or what we will refer to as domains should be included. Depending upon the venue, purpose and the professional discipline, conducting the assessment, these domains may change slightly. These domains will be briefly discussed with suggestions for the use of potential assessment instruments.

Assessment of Physical Functioning–This consists of the assessment of one's ability to perform activities of daily living (ADLs) and instrumental activities of daily living (IADLs). The assessment of function serves to provide a baseline for future comparisons of function, determine the need for services as well as technology aids, and can be used as eligibility criteria for services (such as in the case of Medicaid waiver programs). A variety of measures such as the Katz Index of Independence in Activities of Daily Living, the Barthel Index and the Functional Independence Measure are commonly used. An extensive discussion of various measures of function has been published elsewhere (Emlet, Crabtree, Condon, & Treml, 1996; Pearson, 2000).

Assessment of Emotions and Cognitive Function–Because of the prevalence of psychiatric disorders in old age, a psychosocial assessment should screen for potential cognitive and affective disorders (Emlet, Crabtree, Condon, & Treml, 1996). Mental status assessments are pivotal in evaluating older adults in order to detect unsuspected cognitive impairment (Gallo, Fulmer, Paveza, & Reichel, 2000). Initial assessments of cognitive function typically include questions that assess memory, orientation, and other cognitive abilities in order to identify obvious deficits consistent with dementia (Zarit, 1997). The Mini Mental State Exam (MMSE) (Folstein, Folstein, and McHugh, 1975) is considered the most commonly used quantitative instrument for screening of moderate to severe dementia (Chodosh, 2000). Depression in older adults often goes unrecognized and can have serious consequences if left untreated. Self-report instruments such as the Geriatric Depression Scale [GDS] (Yesavage, Brink, Rose, Lum, Huang, Adey, & Leirer, 1983) are common methods for initial assessments. The Center for Epidemiological Studies Depression Scale [CES-D] (Radloff, 1977) is another self-report assessment instrument for depression. The CES-D has been found to have "acceptable properties for use as a screening instrument for major depression in older primary care patients" (Lyness et al., 1997, p. 452).

Social Support–The assessment of social support networks in the lives of older persons are important for several reasons including: determining if they have the social resources (including social support and social network) to remain living independently in the community; and to identify individuals who are isolated and vulnerable (lacking social support) (Levin, 2000). Antonucci and colleagues (1997) suggests that such an assessment will help identify others who might be available to perform critical tasks, i.e., help with medications, transportation or personal care. While some instruments provide a quantitative account of social support, such as the Lubben Social Network Scale (Lubben, Lee, & Gironda, 2000), others such as the Hierarchical Mapping Technique (Antonucci, 1986) provides a more qualitative method of assessment.

Sexual Health–Sexuality is too often overlooked in the process of conducting heath assessments with older adults because of stereotypical beliefs about aging and sexuality. Key components of taking a sexual history should include the older person's normal sexual patterns, changes that have transpired due to aging or loss of partners and possible problems with sexual functioning associated with medications (Gallo, Fulmer, Paveza & Reichel, 2000). As will be discussed later in more detail, sexual practices such as unsafe intercourse should be examined closely and not overlooked due to ageist beliefs.

Spirituality–The integration of a spiritual assessment has been said to "be a key feature to understanding the overall well-being of an older adult" (Gallo, Fulmer, Paveza, & Reichel, 2000, p. 184). The inclusion of spirituality and religion is important as older people make up a large part of those who attend church or other formal religious gatherings. Religion and spirituality have been associated with various benefits including positive outcomes in social functioning and psychological well-being (Olson & Kane, 2000) and improved coping with end-of-life issues (Liefer, 1996). Various means of defining and assessing spirituality have been developed. The Brief Multidimensional Measure of Religiousness and Spirituality encompasses 12 domains of religion and spirituality, including: daily spiritual experiences, values/beliefs, forgiveness, private religious practices, religious and spiritual coping, religious support, religious/spiritual history, commitment, organizational religiousness and religious preferences (Fetzer Institute, 1999). Recently, Hodge (2001) developed an Interpretive Anthropological Framework, defined as a "multidimensional framework for understanding the personal subjective reality of spiritually in clients' lives" (p. 208). This qualitative framework examines various aspects of the "spiritual" and includes affect, behavior, cognition, communication, conscience, and intuition.

Medications–The use of prescription and over-the-counter (OTC) medications is overrepresented in older adults. Older adults use approximately 30% of all prescription medications and 40% of OTC medications (National Council on Patient Information and Education, 2002). On average, older persons use 4.5 different prescription medications in addition to OTC products, making polypharmacy a critical issue for older persons (Gallo, Fulmer, Paveza, & Reichel, 2000). Non-adherence to medications has been estimated at 50% (Schaffer & Yoon, 2001). Thus, a thorough inventory and evaluation of medications is an important element in the assessment of older persons.

Caregiver Health and Burden–Family caregiving is defined as providing, arranging or overseeing services that an older persons needs due to functional disability or health needs (Gaugler, Kane, & Langlois, 2000). Family members play a key role in helping disabled elders remain at home. Data from the Agency for Healthcare Research and Quality (2000) indicates that 79% of those who need long term care live at home or in the community rather than an institution. Excessive and unchecked caregiver burden, however, may increase the potential for elder abuse and out-of-home placement. Since relatives and spouses commit the majority of domestic elder abuse (National Center for Elder Abuse, 1998) the assessment of caregiver burden is essential. Various caregiver assessment instruments been developed for disease specific (i.e., Alzheimer's disease) and non-disease specific situations. Reviews of these instruments can be found elsewhere (Gaugler, Kane, & Langlois, 2000; Emlet, Crabtree, Condon, & Treml, 1996).

Assessment in HIV/AIDS

When working with persons living with HIV/AIDS, a thorough assessment of needs is also necessary. As stated by Wright (2000), through the assessment of all aspects of a person's life "social workers are better prepared to create environments what will increase a person's understanding and, thus, strengthen their ability to adapt and cope with this [HIV/AIDS] complex process" (p. 19). Gallego (1998) reminds us that in working with individuals with HIV disease, the assessment process may need to be conducted over time and will be successfully completed after establishing mutual trust and rapport.

This section will review the areas of assessment covered previously as they relate to HIV disease. Additional areas of assessment will be discussed as appropriate that are idiosyncratic to the assessment process with HIV/AIDS.

Assessment of Physical Functioning–Although the actual process of ADLs and IADLs do not differ significantly from one disease process to another, the context does change. In working with older adults, barring an acute episode such as a stroke, changes in ADL and IADL dependence is often gradual. HIV disease, however, is different. As Giulino (1998) states, "the illness has an unpredictable course and medically affects patients in different ways; thus determining the timing or the severity of the symptoms is difficult" (pp. 165-166). Babcock (1998) provides an example in which an individual diagnosed with AIDS goes from moderate dependence in ADLs to the need for 24-hour assistance in a period of two to four weeks. Multiple factors can affect one's functional dependence including: generalized weakness, opportunistic infections, AIDS related neuropsychiatric disorders, medication side-effects or any combination of factors (Wyatt, 1996). Despite the advances in antiretroviral therapy, people continue to become quite ill and die from AIDS. An examination of data from the CDC indicates that from June of 1999 through June of 2001 over 37,000 individuals of all ages died from AIDS in the United States alone (CDC, 2000, 2002). Assessment of ADL function in this population needs to be done consistently and reliably.

Assessment of Emotions and Cognitive Function–Cognitive and emotional issues can significantly impact the lives of people with HIV disease. Leavitt (2000) suggests a continuum of symptomatology, including preexisting mental illness, mental health issue arising from HIV related stressors and psychiatric/organic problems. Major depressive disorder and other forms of depression have been found to be more prevalent among HIV infected individuals than the general population (Hinkin, Castellon, Atkinson, & Goodkin, (2001). Self-report and structured clinical rating scales have been used extensively in identifying depression in persons living with HIV (Hinkin, Castellon, Atkinson, & Goodkin, (2001). Wu and colleagues (1991) have identified 30 items from the Medical Outcome Study (MOS) and found questions to be reliable in identifying a number of clinical issues including depression in persons with HIV disease.

A critical component of assessment is the identification of cognitive impairment related to HIV. Cognitive impairment increases as an individual becomes more immune compromised and symptomatic (Buckingham, 1998). Goodkin et al. (2001) delineates two identifiable conditions, minor cognitive motor disorder (MCMD) and HIV-1-associated dementia (HAD). These conditions involve information processing, speed, memory, attention, abstraction executive function and motor abilities. Because the most prominent feature at initial presentation is slowing of movements and thinking (Buckingham, 1998), symptoms are often missed as HIV dementia is subcortical rather than cortical (such as with Alzheimer's disease) and standard mental status exams do not always identify early symptoms. Knippels, Goodkin, Weiss, Wilkie, and Antoni (2002) found the four questions which make up the cognitive functional status subscale of the MOS to be significantly associated with results of neuropsychological testing in the identification of HIV-related cognitive symptoms.

Social Support–The assessment of social support for persons with HIV/AIDS is similar to that of older persons. At the same time, however, important differences in the source of support and the function of that support have been found. Sexual orientation has been shown to alter sources of identified social support. Beeler and colleagues (1999) found friendship networks to be among the most important sources of social support for midlife and older lesbian and gays. In a study of gay men with HIV, Kadushin (1999) found the involvement of family differed at various stages of HIV disease. She found that once an individual had a diagnosis of AIDS and needed increased care, these men received significantly higher levels of support from their families than those with HIV. Linsk and Bonk (2000) remind us that while "family and friends are generally the chief sources of support . . . our notion of family must be expanded to incorporate the most important individuals as defined by the client" (p. 219).

Sexual Health–HIV assessment must explore the client's norms, values and beliefs about sexual behavior. Attitudes about HIV transmission, factors associated with risk and barriers to risk reduction and sexual self-efficacy/self-esteems are areas that need exploration (Wright, 2000). Questions should include information about sexual partners, types of protection used (including folk methods), history of forced sex and sexual activity related to substance abuse. Ellenberg (1998) provides an extensive framework for initiating a sexual history.

Spirituality–As with older adults, spirituality is often important in the lives of people with HIV disease. Feelings of spirituality may be long-standing or may be triggered by learning of having a life-threatening disease. People may attempt to reconnect to religious traditions from the past or turn to philosophies or religions new to them (Poindexter, 2000). One important consideration is that some religious traditions have held harsh judgments about drug use, homosexuality or addiction, causing persons with HIV to feel discouraged about seeking out support from religious organizations (Brennan, 1998). Social workers and other health professionals need to become comfortable listening to the spiritual concerns of clients without imposing our own religious views and beliefs (Poindexter, 2000). It is helpful to ask clients about their spiritual and religious beliefs, helping them understand the important difference. Having an understanding of where to access spiritual resources that are HIV sensitive can be of great help.

Immune Function–Any person diagnosed with HIV is immediately confronted with a new vocabulary. To know you are HIV+ is not enough information. Osmond (1998) suggests that the CD4 (t-cell) count is perhaps the most important measurable marker of disease progression for HIV. CD4 cells or lymphocytes are instrumental in immune reactions (Casey, Cohen, & Hughes, 1996). Normal CD4 counts range from 500-1000 mm^3. The CD4 cell is the target of the human immunodeficiency virus, which it infects. The virus takes over the cell's "powerhouse" to produce more viral copies and thus depletes the store of CD4 cells. As the number of CD4 cells decline, the body becomes less able to maintain immunity against microorganisms that is was previously exposed to (tuberculosis and toxoplasmosis are examples of this). The relationship between specific CD4 values and opportunistic infections as well as other medical complications has been well documented (Bartlett, 2001; Casey, Cohen, & Hughes, 1996). People infected with HIV and with CD4 values less than 200 per mm^3 frequently experience pneumonias, lymphomas, Herpes zoster, and other diseases. Many of these infections are AIDS defining. As of 1993, a documented CD4 count of < 200 cells per mm^3 itself is an AIDS-defining condition (Casey, 1996). Quantitative plasma HIV RNA testing has revolutionized the monitoring of HIV disease and treatment. This value, known as *viral load* provides clinicians with a measurement of the actual number of viral copies in a volume of blood. Values can range from "undetectable" to several million. The undetectability of virus in the plasma, however, does not mean that there is no virus in the body. Latent reservoirs retain HIV in a form that can be quickly circulated in the presence of treatment failure or discontinuance (Liegler, 2001). The monitoring of the viral load can provide valuable information to the patient and clinician and is now considered to be a primary marker for treatment decisions (Osmond, 1998). A surge in the viral load in a patient on highly active antiretroviral medications (HAART) can signal viral resistance to components of therapy, adherence issues, or laboratory errors. Liegler (2001) suggests that "viral load during long-term therapy is of less clear prognostic significance" (p. 9), suggesting other factors, including serial CD4 counts and clinical symptoms must be taken into account.

Disclosure and Confidentiality–Individuals who have HIV/AIDS are faced with the possibility of rejection, betrayal, and discrimination following disclosure of their diagnosis (Poindexter, 2000). Gallego (1998) reminds us that many women are afraid of revealing their HIV status in fear of losing their support systems. Each individual is faced with the decision of who to tell and when to tell. As part of the assessment process, it is important to inquire about whom the client has shared their HIV status with, including immediate biological family, extended network of family and friends and health care providers. Additionally it may be helpful to know for example, if people at the worksite, including the boss or supervisor has been told (Giulino, 1998)? For individuals who do not commonly work in the HIV arena, it is critical to remember that confidentiality respects the right of the client to make decisions about where and with whom this information is shared (Giddens, Ka'opua & Tomaszewski, 2000). A well intentioned act as subtle as mailing written information about HIV to a client's home when the client has not disclosed their status to all family members can be a potential breach of confidentiality.

Caregiver Health and Burden–Caregivers of persons living with HIV/ AIDS face a multitude of challenges. These challenges will depend upon the nature of the relationship prior to taking on the caregiving role and the level of disability of the care receiver. Several issues are likely to exist for most caregivers. The caregiver will experience role change. As Gordon-Garofalo (2000) states, "the caregiver becomes counselor, advisor, sounding board, decision maker, nurse, companion and lover to the PLWA" (p. 110). The caregiver will also face issues of commitment to the care receiver. In circumstance where infidelity has occurred, this may be a substantial obstacle. Multiple losses will multiply throughout the course of the illness and may include personal time, dreams and plans, lifestyle and changes in relationship. Additionally, stigma and isolation may occur through "courtesy stigma" (Goffman, 1963) which is ascribed to those voluntarily attached to a stigmatized group.

ASSESSING OLDER ADULTS WITH HIV/AIDS: PUTTING IT ALL TOGETHER

Older adults who have been diagnosed with HIV/AIDS or at-risk for infection involve the intersection of two different populations, each with its own unique issues, concerns, and culture. In providing assessment services to this population, it is necessary, therefore, to include important elements that recognize the needs of both populations, combine those elements when necessary and understand where complications and contradictions occur. Table 3 provides a format in which to examine the areas of integration as well as potential contradictions or complications.

The assessment of physical functioning is of great importance in working with older adults who have been diagnosed with HIV disease. It is important to recall that the changes in physical function may change more rapidly with HIV disease than with many of the chronic

TABLE 3. Assessment Domains for Specific and Combined Populations

Domain	Older Adults	Persons Living with HIV/AIDS	Older Persons With HIV/AIDS
Physical Functioning	✓	✓	Comorbidity may result in decline in functioning from various sources. Functioning may decline more rapidly and more sporadically with HIV disease than typical chronic diseases associated with aging.
Cognitive/Affective	✓	✓	Cognitive decline in older adults may be due to a variety of factors including dementias normally associated with aging in addition to HIV dementia. Initial symptoms of HIV-related cognitive decline may not be found using traditional mental status exams often used with older adults.
Social Support	✓	✓	Older adults with HIV/AIDS, depending upon their history, may have limited contact with biological family. Additionally, social supports common to younger persons with HIV, such as parents and even siblings, may be unavailable to older adults due to death or frailty of family members.
Sexual Health	✓	✓	Taking sexual histories with older adults requires an understanding of cohort terminology and may require altering language typically used with younger clients. Ageist attitudes among professionals about sexuality must be recognized.
Spirituality	✓	✓	Older adults may need assistance with disclosing diagnosis to clergy or may need to locate spiritual resources that are HIV sensitive. Individuals may have broken ties with religious organizations from the past who engaged in "blaming" behaviors.
Immune Function	✓	✓	Senescence of the immune system (aging process) may serve to accelerate the decline of CD4 t-cells that are diminished through HIV. Older adults will need to be educated about the importance of CD4 and viral load and may need to be assisted with regular and ongoing testing.
Disclosure	✓	✓	Determine whom the client has disclosed their HIV status to. This should include various family members, friends, health care providers, clergy, as well as individuals from the client job (if working).
Caregiver Well-Being	✓	✓	Caregivers of individuals with HIV may suffer from many of the same physical, emotional, financial, and social burdens of other caregivers. In addition, associative stigma may exist, depending upon the disclosure of the care receiver's HIV status.

diseases associated with aging. The issue of comorbdity, however, is of great importance. An older adult's physical function may be impacted not only by HIV, but by aging related diseases such as arthritis, non-HIV related respiratory or cardiac disease or other disease processes. Skeist and Keiser (1997) found persons age 55 and over to have significantly higher rates of concurrent non HIV-related health conditions than their younger counterparts. In these instances, it may be necessary to reassess ADL and IADL function more frequency in order to ascertain sudden changes in status.

The assessment of cognitive changes in this population is complicated by the intersection of aging and HIV. Changes in cognitive status must be considered in the context of potential disease processes commonly associated with aging (such as Alzheimer's disease) in addition to HIV associated cognitive changes. There is some evidence to suggest that HIV-dementia as an AIDS defining illness may be more common in older adults (Inungu, Mokotoff, & Kent, 2001). It is important to consider that AIDS related dementia is characterized by a rapid progression and is more often associated with peripheral neuropathies, myelopathies, and general physical complaints such as weight loss and fatigue than the cortical dementias (Chiao, Ries, & Sande, 1999). In these circumstances, the use of the functional status subscale of the MOS may be added to cognitive testing typically done with older adults in order to capture the more subtle symptoms associated with HIV related dementia.

As suggested in Table 3, the social support networks of older adults with HIV disease may differ in several ways. First, the size of the network may be compromised due to loss and death as compared to younger adults. Parents of older adults are often deceased or too ill to provide assistance. Friends and family may also be unavailable. Instances have been documented where older adults have been ostracized by friends and adult children due to their HIV status (Bressler, 1987; Kadushin, 1999). Depending upon other factors such as sexual orientation, the social support network of older adults may also be non-traditional, drawing more upon "fictive kin" and friends than biological family. It is important to keep in mind that many gay and lesbian older adults had not come out for many years, maintaining heterosexual relationships during their younger adult lives.

The assessment of sexual practices and history is critical to all individuals with HIV disease. Data on the increased frequency of "unknown" risk among older adults (CDC, 1998; Inungu, Mokotoff, & Kent, 2001) suggests that one's understanding of risk behavior or willingness to discuss those behaviors may be impacted by age. Depending upon the history and sexual orientation of the older adult, social workers and other health professionals may need to alter their language in conducting sexual histories. Many of the individuals of concern grew up or were young adults during World War II. This generation is familiar with the terms of *venereal disease* and can understand that vernacular. Additionally, while younger adults may be used to hearing more explicit language related to sexual practices, some older adults may be embarrassed or insulted by such language. In taking sexual histories with older adults, awareness of personally held ageist stereotypes by the assessor is important to bring to consciousness. Language may need to be adjusted or altered for older individuals. Genke (2000) and Emlet (1997) both provide questions for use in the sexual histories of older adults that have been suggested by the National Association on HIV Over Fifty (NAHOF).

The area of spirituality and religion may serve as a major contradiction for older persons with HIV/AIDS as well as a means of comfort. While religion and spirituality may be of great importance to many older persons, those very social institutions have often caused conflict for the individual. For example, many gay men have been labeled sinners by those institutions and excluded from various activities (Anderson, 1996). Older adults may need assistance with disclosing their status to clergy or may need help in locating HIV sensitive spiritual support.

Recent research has suggested that older adults are prescribed antiretroviral therapy at equal proportions to their younger counterparts (Emlet & Berghuis, 2002; Wellons et al., 2002) and that those therapies are equally as effective (Wellons et al., 2002). Older adults may need additional assistance in understanding the processes in determining virology, i.e., CD4 count and viral load. When necessary, professional (non-HIV savvy) staff working with an older adult with HIV may need to seek out consultation to better understand the terminology used in virology.

Caregivers of adults or children with HIV disease face many of the same emotional and physical challenges as caregivers of individuals with other illnesses. HIV caregivers are often older themselves and face their own aging related limitation, and may suffer from "grief overload" (Poindexter & Linsk, 2000) caused by multiple HIV-related losses. Additionally, HIV affected caregivers may experience associative stigma (Poindexter, 1999). Poindexter points out, caregivers who experience stigma from their social networks and society as a whole may respond by "withdrawing from or ignoring their own social needs and become further isolated" (p. 49).

CONCLUSION

Older adults will continue to be infected with and affected by HIV in the coming years. As this paper has suggested, these individuals face the same problems and issues of their non-HIV infected peers. At the same time, however, additional issues and complications exist that makes working with older adults with HIV/AIDS a challenge for social workers, nurses and other health professionals from a variety of health care and social venues. It was the intention of the authors to present to the reader an overview of the issues faced by this emerging vulnerable population while providing a systematic examination of the factors associated with a comprehensive and skillful assessment of the needs of these individuals.

AUTHOR NOTE

The first author wishes to acknowledge the support received from the John A. Hartford Foundation through the Hartford Geriatric Social Work Faculty Scholars Program in preparing this manuscript.

REFERENCES

Agency for Healthcare Research and Quality (2000). *Long-term Care Users Range in Age and Most Do Not Live in Nursing Homes: Research Alert.* Rockville, MD : Agency for Healthcare Research and Quality.

AIDS Action Council (June 2001). Older Americans and HIV. *The Body: An AIDS and HIV information resource.* Retrieved June 18, 2002, from *http://www.thebody.com/aac/brochures/older_americans.html.*

Anderson, G. (1996). The older gay man. In K. M. Nokes (ed.). *HIV/AIDS and the older adult* (pp. 63-79. Bristol, PA: Taylor and Francis.

Antonucci, T.C. (1986). Hierarchical mapping technique: Measuring social support networks. *Generations, 10*(4), 10-12.

Antonucci, T. C., Sherman, A. M., & Vandewater, E. A. (1997). Measures of social support and caregiver burden. *Generations, 21* (1), 48-51.

Babcock, J. H. (1998). Bereavement work in the acute care setting. In D. M Aronstein & B. J. Thompson (eds.). *HIV and social work: A practitioner's guide* (pp. 109-122). New York: Haworth Press.

Bartlett, J. (2001). *2001-2002 Medical Management of HIV Infection.* Baltimore, MD: Johns Hopkins University, Division of Infectious Diseases.

Beeler, J. A., Rawls, T. D., Herdt, G., & Cohler, B. J. (1999). The needs of older lesbians and gay men in Chicago. *Journal of Gay and Lesbian Social Services, 9*(1), 31-49.

Brennan, D. J. (1998). Bereavement work in hospice and home care. In D. M Aronstein & B. J. Thompson (eds.). *HIV and social work: A practitioner's guide* (pp. 135-144). New York: The Haworth Press, Inc.

Bressler, J. (1987). HIV infected elders. *Generations, 13*, 45-47.

Buckingham, S. L. (1998). Identifying and treating HIV-associated dementia. In D. M. Aronstein & B. J. Thompson (eds.). *HIV and social work: A practitioner's guide* (pp. 281-291). New York: The Haworth Press, Inc.

Casey, K.M., Cohen, F., & Hughes, A. (1996). *Association of Nurses in AIDS Care Core Curriculum for HIV/AIDS Nursing*, Philadelphia: NurseCom Inc.

Centers for Disease Control and Prevention (1998). AIDS among persons aged > 50 years–United States, 1991-1996. *Morbidity and Mortality Weekly Report, 47*(2), 21-27.

Centers for Disease Control and Prevention (2000). *HIV/AIDS Surveillance Report Mid-Year Edition, 11*(1).

Centers for Disease Control and Prevention (2002). *HIV/AIDS Surveillance Report Mid-Year Edition, 13*(1).

Chiao, E.Y., Ries, K.M., and Sande, M.A. (1999). AIDS and the elderly. *Clinical Infectious Disease, 28*, 740-745.

Chodosh, J. (2000). Cognitive screening tests: Mini mental state exam. In M. D. Mezey (ed.). *The encyclopedia of elder care: The comprehensive resource on geriatric and social care* (pp. 142-144). New York: Springer.

Ellenberg, L. W. (1998). HIV risk assessment in mental health settings. In D. M Aronstein & B. J. Thompson (eds.). *HIV and social work: A practitioner's guide* (pp. 232-246). New York: The Haworth Press, Inc.

Emlet, C. A., (1997). HIV/AIDS in the elderly: A hidden population. *Home Care Provider, 2*, 69-75.

Emlet, C. A., & Berghuis, J. P. (in press). Service Priorities, Use and Needs: Views of Older and Younger Consumers living with HIV/AIDS. *Journal of Mental Health and Aging, 8*(4).

Emlet, C., Crabtree, J., Condon, V., & Treml, L. (1996). *In home assessment of older adults: An interdisciplinary approach*. Gaithersburg, MD: Aspen.

Emlet, C. A., & Farkas, K. J. (2002). Correlates of service utilization among midlife and older adults with HIV/AIDS: The role of age in the equation. *Journal of Aging and Health, 14*, 315-335.

Emlet, C. A., & Poindexter, C. C. (2002). *The unserved, unseen and unheard: Integrating program for HIV-infected and affected elders*. Manuscript under review.

Emlet, C.A., Tangenberg, K., and Siverson, C. (2002). A feminist approach to practice in working with mid-life and older women with HIV/AIDS. *Affilia: Journal of Women and Social Work, 17*, 229-251.

Ferro, S. & Salit, I. E. (1992). HIV infection in patients over 55 years of age. *Journal of Acquired Immune Deficiency Syndrome, 5*, 348-355.

Fetzer Institute (1999). *Multidimensional measurement of religiousness/spirituality for use in health research*. Kalamazoo, MI: Author.

Folstein, M.F., Folstein, S.E., & McHugh, P.R. (1975). "Mini-Mental State": A practical method for grading the cognitive state of patients for the clinician. *Journal of Psychiatric Research, 12*, 189-198.

Fowler, J.P. (1999). HIV in people over 50. *Focus: A Guide to AIDS Research and Counseling, 14*(9), 1-4.

Gallego, S. M. (1998). Providing services to HIV-Positive women. In D. M Aronstein & B. J. Thompson (eds.). *HIV and social work: A practitioner's guide* (pp. 431-442). New York: The Haworth Press, Inc.

Gallo, J.J., Fulmer, T., Paveza, G. J., & Reichel, W. (2000). *Handbook of geriatric assessment* (3rd ed). Gaithersburg, MD: Aspen.

Gaugler, J. E., Kane, R. A., & Langlois, J. (2000). Assessment of family caregivers of older adults. In R. L. Kane & R. A. Kane (eds.). *Assessing older persons: Measures, meaning and practical applications* (pp. 320-359). New York: Oxford University Press.

Genke, J. (2000). HIV/AIDS and older adults: The invisible ten percent. *Care Management Journals, 2*(3), 196-205.

Geron, S. M. (1997). Introduction: Taking the measure of assessment. *Generations, 21*(1), 5-9.

Giddens, B., Ka'opua, L., & Tomaszewski, E. (2000). Ethical issues and dilemmas in HIV/AIDS. In V. J. Lynch (ed.). *HIV/AIDS at year 2000: A sourcebook for social workers* (pp. 33-49). Boston: Allyn and Bacon.

Giulino, P. U. (1998). Individual clinical issues. In D. M Aronstein & B. J. Thompson (eds.). *HIV and social work: A practitioner's guide* (pp. 165-181). New York: Haworth Press.

Goffman, E. (1963). *Stigma: Notes on the management of spoiled identity*. Englewood Cliffs, NJ: Prentice Hall.

Goodkin, K., Wilkie, F. L., Concha, M., Hinkin, C. H., Symes, S., & Baldewicz, T. T. et al. (2001). Aging and neuro-AIDS conditions and the changing spectrum of HIV-1-associated morbidity and mortality. *Journal of Clinical Epidemiology, 54*, S35-S43.

Gordon-Garofalo, V. (2000). Social work treatment with caregivers. In V. J. Lynch (ed.). *HIV/AIDS at year 2000: A sourcebook for social workers* (pp. 107-122). Boston: Allyn and Bacon.

Heckman, T.G., Heckman, B.D., Kochman, A., Sikkema, K.J., Suhr, J., & Goodkin, K. (2002). Psychological symptoms among persons 50 years of age and older living with HIV disease. *Aging & Mental Health, 6*(2), 121-128.

Heckman, T.G., Kochman, A., Sikkema, K.J., and Kalichman, S.C. (1999). Depressive symptomatology, daily stressors, and ways of coping among middle-age and older adults living with HIV disease. *Journal of Mental Health and Aging, 5*(4), 1-11.

Hinkin, C. H., Castellon, S. A., Atkinson, J. H., & Goodkin, K. (2001). Neuropsychiatric aspects of HIV infection among older adults. *Journal of Clinical Epidemiology, 54*, S44-S52.

Hodge, D. R. (2001). Spiritual assessment: A review of major qualitative methods and a new framework for assessing spirituality. *Social Work, 46*, 203-214.

Inungu, J. N., Mokotoff, E. D., & Kent, J. B. (2001). Characteristics of HIV infection in patients fifty year or older in Michigan. *AIDS Patient Care and STDs, 15*, 567-573.

Johnson, M., Haight, B.D., Faan, P.H., and Benedict, S. (1998). AIDS in older people: A literature review for clinical nursing research and practice. *Journal of Gerontological Nursing, 24*(4), 8-13.

Kadushin, G. (1999). Barriers to social support and support received from their families or origin among gay men with HIV/AIDS. *Health and Social Work, 24,* 198-209.

Knippels, H. M. A., Goodkin, K., Weiss, J. J., Wilkie, F. L., & Antoni, M. H. (2002). The importance of cognitive self-report in early HIV-1 infection: Validation of a cognitive functional status subscale. *AIDS, 16,* 259-267.

Leavitt, E. (2000). Mental health issues in HIV disease. In V. J. Lynch (ed.). *HIV/AIDS at year 2000: A sourcebook for social workers* (pp. 228-241). Boston: Allyn and Bacon.

Levin, C. (2000). Social functioning. In R. L Kane and R. A. Kane (eds.). *Assessing older persons: Measures, meaning and practical applications* (pp. 170-199). New York: Oxford University Press.

Liefer, R. (1996). Psychological and spiritual factors in chronic illness. *American Behavioral Scientist, 39,* 752-766.

Liegler, T., & Grant, R. (2001). HIV Viral Load Assay. HIV Insite Knowledge Base. University of California, San Francisco [online]. Retrieved June 21, 2002 from: *http://hivinsite.org/InSite.jsp?page=kb-02&doc=kb-02-02-02-01*

Linsk, N.L. (2000). HIV among older adults: Age-specific issues in prevention and treatment. *The AIDS reader, 10*(7), 430-440.

Linsk, N. L., & Bonk, N. (2000). Adherence to treatment as social work challenges. In V. J. Lynch (ed.). *HIV/AIDS at year 2000: A sourcebook for social workers* (pp. 211-227). Boston: Allyn and Bacon.

Lubben, J., Lee, A., & Gironda, M. (2000, May). *Analysis and further development of the Lubben Social Network Scale.* Presented at the ESRC Seminar Series, Social Networks and Social Exclusion, University of Wales, Bangor.

Lyness, J. M., Noel, T. K., Cox, C., King, D. A., Conwell, Y., & Caine, E. D. (1997). Screening for depression in elderly primary care patients: A comparison of the Center for Epidemiologic Studies-Depression Scale and the Geriatric Depression Scale. *Archives of Internal Medicine, 157,* 449-454.

National Center on Elder Abuse (1998). *National elder abuse incidence study: Final Report.* Washington, DC: American Public Human Services Association.

National Council on Patient Information and Education (2002). Older adults. Retrieved June, 18, 2002 from *http://www.talkaboutrx.org/select.html#old.*

Olson, D. M., & Kane, R. A. (2000). Spiritual assessment. In R. L. Kane and R. A. Kane (eds.), *Assessing older persons: Measures, meaning and practical applications* (pp.300-319). New York: Oxford University Press.

Osmond, D. (1998). Epidemiology of disease progression in HIV. HIV Insite Knowledge Base. University of California, San Francisco [online]. Retrieved June 21, 2002 from: *http://hivinsite.org/InSite.jsp?page=kb-03&doc=kb-03-01-04*

Pearson, V. I. (2000). Assessment of function in older adults. In R. L. Kane and R. A. Kane (eds.), *Assessing older persons: Measures, meaning and practical applications* (pp.17-48). New York: Oxford University Press.

Poindexter, C. C., & Linsk, N. L. (1999). HIV-related stigma in a sample of HIV-affected older female African American caregivers. *Social Work, 44,* 49-61.

Poindexter, C. C., (2000). Common concerns: Social and psychological issues for persons with HIV. In V. J. Lynch (ed.). *HIV/AIDS at year 2000: A sourcebook for social workers* (pp. 18-31). Boston: Allyn and Bacon.

Poindexter, C. C., & Linsk, N. L. (2000). HIV and later life. In V. J. Lynch (ed.). *HIV/AIDS at year 2000: A sourcebook for social workers* (pp. 138-147). Boston: Allyn and Bacon.

Radloff, L. S. (1977). The CES-D Scale: A self-report depression scale for research in the general population. *Applied Psychological Measurement, 1*(3), 385-401.

Rubenstein, L.Z. (1987). Geriatric assessment: An overview of its impacts. *Clinics in Geriatric Medicine, 3*(1), 1-15.

Schaffer, S. D., & Yoon, S. L. (2001). Evidence-based methods to enhance medication adherence. *The Nurse Practitioner, 26*(12), 44, 50, 52 & 54.

Skeist, D. J., & Keiser, P. (1997). Human immunodeficiency virus infection in patients older than 50 years. *Archives of Family Medicine, 6*(3), 289-294.

Szirony, T.A. (1999). Infection with HIV in the elderly population. *Journal of Gerontological Nursing, 25*(10), 25-31.

Urdangarin, C. F. (2000). Comprehensive geriatric assessment and management. In R. L. Kane and R. A. Kane (eds.), *Assessing older persons: Measures, meaning and practical applications* (pp. 383-405). New York: Oxford University Press.

Wellons, M. F., Sanders, L., Edwards, L. J., Bartlett, J. A., Heald, A. E., & Schmader, K. E. (2002). HIV infection: Treatment outcomes in older and younger adults. *Journal of the American Geriatrics Society, 50*, 603-607.

Wooten-Bielski, K. (1999). HIV & AIDS in older adults. *Geriatric Nursing, 20*(5), 268-272.

Wright, E. M. (2000). The psychosocial context. In V. J. Lynch (ed.). *HIV/AIDS at year 2000: A sourcebook for social workers* (pp. 18-31). Boston: Allyn and Bacon.

Wu, A. W., Rubin, H. R., Mathews, W. C., Ware, J. E. et al. (1991). A health status questionnaire using 30 items from the Medical Outcome Study: Preliminary validation in persons with early HIV infection. *Medical Care, 29*, 786-798.

Wyatt, A. (1996). Long-term care. In K. M. Nokes (ed.). *HIV/AIDS and the older adult* (pp. 81-94). Bristol, PA: Taylor and Francis.

Yesavage, J.A., Brink, T.L., Rose, T.L., Lum, O., Huang, V., Adey, M., & Leirer, V.O. (1983). Development and validation of a geriatric depression screening scale: A preliminary report. *Journal of Psychiatric Research, 17*, 37-49.

Zarit, S. H. (1997). Brief measures of depression and cognitive function. *Generations, 21*(1), 41-43.

Zelenetz, P.D., & Epstein, M.E. (1998). HIV in the elderly. *AIDS Patient Care and STD's, 12*(4), 255-262.

P.S. I Love You:
Long-Distance Caregiving

Beverly B. Koerin, PhD, MSW

Marcia P. Harrigan, PhD, MSW

SUMMARY. Family caregiving plays an important role in our health care delivery system, especially for the frail elderly. Despite a substantial literature on caregiving, there is little research on long-distance caregivers, a population expected to double in the next decade. This paper reports a secondary analysis of data from the 1997 NAC/AARP national survey and focuses on long-distance caregivers. Findings include caregiver and care receiver characteristics, patterns of caregiving, and impacts on caregivers. The data are compared to previous national studies on caregiving and implications for practice and further research are considered. *[Article copies available for a fee from The Haworth Document Delivery Service: 1-800-HAWORTH. E-mail address: <docdelivery@haworthpress.com> Website: <http://www.HaworthPress.com> © 2002 by The Haworth Press, Inc. All rights reserved.]*

Beverly B. Koerin is Associate Professor at the School of Social Work, Virginia Commonwealth University, 1001 West Franklin Street, Richmond, VA 23284-2027. Marcia P. Harrigan is Associate Professor and MSW Program Director, School of Social Work, Virginia Commonwealth University, 1001 West Franklin Street, Richmond, VA 23284-2027.

The authors wish to acknowledge NAC and AARP for access to the original data set used in this study.

[Haworth co-indexing entry note]: "P.S. I Love You: Long-Distance Caregiving." Koerin, Beverly B., and Marcia P. Harrigan. Co-published simultaneously in *Journal of Gerontological Social Work* (The Haworth Social Work Practice Press, an imprint of The Haworth Press, Inc.) Vol. 40, No. 1/2, 2002, pp. 63-81; and: *Older People and Their Caregivers Across the Spectrum of Care* (ed: Judith L. Howe) The Haworth Social Work Practice Press, an imprint of The Haworth Press, Inc., 2003, pp. 63-81. Single or multiple copies of this article are available for a fee from The Haworth Document Delivery Service [1-800-HAWORTH, 9:00 a.m. - 5:00 p.m. (EST). E-mail address: docdelivery@haworthpress.com].

KEYWORDS. Caregivers, long-distance, elderly, caregiving, family caregiving, care network

Family caregivers play "an invisible role . . . in our health care delivery system," especially for frail elderly individuals. Over 80% of all home-based care is provided on an informal, unpaid basis by family and friends (National Family Caregivers Association, 2000, p. 2). A 1997 study by the National Alliance for Caregiving (NAC) and the American Association of Retired Persons (AARP) found that over 23% of households in the United States contained at least one individual providing care for a relative or friend aged 50 or older. Many factors have contributed to the growing interest in caregiving. Managed care restrictions on hospital care and home health services have increased demands on family caregivers. Demographic changes (e.g., declining birth date, increased longevity) and women's increasing workforce participation have decreased the pool of caregivers. Geographic mobility of adult children and retirement-age parents has also affected the pool of *local* family caregivers. A 1997 study by the National Council on Aging (NCOA) reported approximately 7 million individuals were caregivers for relatives, usually parents, living many miles away; the number of long-distance (LD) caregivers was projected to double in the next 15 years (*www.ncoa.org*). The purpose of the present research is to explore the characteristics of long-distance caregivers, including caregiver stress and well being and services used by long-distance caregivers.

LITERATURE REVIEW

Scope of Caregiving and Caregiver Profiles

Caregiving has been variously defined in terms of kinship or relationship of caregiver to care receiver, living arrangements, types of care services provided, intensity or duration of the caregiving role, and age and health status of the care receiver (e.g., Barer & Johnson, 1990; Brody, 1985; George & Gwyther, 1986; Mui, 1995; NAC/AARP, 1997; Penrod, Kane, Kane, & Finch, 1995; Stone, Cafferata, & Sangl, 1987; Toseland & Rossiter, 1996). Consequently, estimates on the scope and nature of the caregiving population also vary, based on these definitions as well as the size and sources of the study samples. In 1987, an AARP/Travelers Foundation study estimated 7 million households involved in caregiving activities for an elder. The definition of caregiver was an adult individual who, currently or within the past 12 months, provided assistance to someone over the age of 50 with at least one ADL and at least two or more Instrumental Activities of Daily Living (IADL), such as managing finances, housework, arranging for services to the care recipient (Wagner, 1997a, p. 1). In 1997 the National Alliance for Caregiving (NAC) and the American Association of Retired Persons (AARP) published findings of its national survey, *Family Caregiving in the U.S.* This study estimated there were 22.4 million caregiving households. Caregiving was defined more generally than in previous studies: "providing unpaid care to a relative or friend who is aged 50 or older to help them take care of themselves" (AARP/NAC, 1997, p. 6).

Comparing the 1987 and 1997 studies, Wagner (1997b) noted some similarities and differences in caregiver profiles. The majority of caregivers were women (75% in 1987; 72% in 1997), who were on average 45 years old and providing care for a parent. The 1997 caregivers were more likely to be employed (64%) than 1987 caregivers (55%) and reported spending less time in caregiving activities. Wagner noted there were fewer reported "primary caregivers" in 1997 (41%) than in 1987 (63%), suggesting that many caregivers provide help to an elder, either with assistance from another sibling or relative or by providing such assistance to a sibling or relative. Previous critiques of the caregiving literature have noted that "secondary caregivers" or members of an informal care network have often been ignored (e.g., Barer & Johnson, 1990; Penrod et al., 1995) Several studies have reported "from one to three secondary helpers in the care network in addition to the primary caregiver" (Penrod et al., 1995, p. 489). Long distance caregivers are likely members of this care network, either as secondary helpers or as primary caregivers when there are no local family or friends available for this role.

Caregiving Costs and Benefits

Caregiving involves benefits and costs that are economic, physical, and socio-emotional in nature. The economic costs of caregiving affect individual families and businesses as well, due to caregiving employees' missing work, shifting to part-time status, or leaving the work force entirely. A major focus of the literature has been on caregiver burden and stress (e.g., Biegel, 1995; Cantor, 1983; Pearlin, Mullan, Semple, & Skaff, 1990; Zarit, Reever, & Bach-Peterson, 1980). Caregiver burden has two dimensions: objective burden refers to the time, efforts, tasks services, and financial supports involved in caregiving that disrupt or change the caregiver's life situation, while subjective burden refers to the caregiver's perceptions, attitudes and emotions about caregiving (Biegel, 1995; Montgomery, Gonyea, & Hooyman, 1985). Caregiver burden negatively impacts the health and well-being of caregivers. While some caregivers experience financial hardships or physical health declines, many studies have documented the pervasiveness of emotional strains (Brody, 1985).

The experience of long-distance caregivers may be different from other caregivers in both objective and subjective dimensions of caregiver burden (Montgomery, Gonyea, & Hooyman, 1985). Experts suggest that "providing care for parents or elderly relatives nearby often is more physically exhausting than long-distance care, while long-distance care often causes more psychological stress" (Wagner, 1997a, p. iii-5).

Long Distance Caregiving

In marked contrast to the substantial research on caregiving, there is little information on the long-distance (LD) caregiver. Most information is found in popular literature sources that provide practical suggestions for long-distance caregivers (e.g., AARP, 1994; Health, 1993; numerous caregiving websites with "long-distance" links). Although rarely defined, LD caregiving has been operationalized in terms of miles or travel time that separate caregiver from care receiver. The National Council on the Aging study defined LD caregivers as those living at least one hour away from the care receiver (Wagner, 1997a). Schoonover, Brody, Hoffman, and Kleban's (1988) study of parent care and "geographically distant children" defined this population as those living "more than 50 miles" from their aging parents, "a threshold point at which visiting and face-to-face interaction between children and elderly parents decreases significantly" (p. 475).

LD caregivers face unique difficulties. First, LD caregiving creates challenges in assessing the needs of the care receiver and knowing when your help is needed. While critical events, such as hospitalizations or accidents, may provide obvious indicators of need, many older adults experience gradual declines in their functioning. Further complicating accurate needs assessment, some aging and/or ailing parents, not wanting to worry their adult children and "Making the most of geographic privacy" (Hooyman & Lustbader, 1986, p. 22), may not disclose their health status or care needs. Conversely, aging parents, neighbors, or local relatives may provide reports that exaggerate the situation. "You need to make sure that what you hear long distance from your parent and about your parent matches the reality of the situation" (Carton, 2000).

Once the need for assistance has been identified, locating services and monitoring them can be problematic, particularly in rural areas where few services exist. The geriatric care manager is described in the literature as an effective way to provide local oversight of services to the care receiver and a solution to difficulties experienced by the LD caregiver (e.g., Weaver, 2001). However, this assumes the local availability of geriatric case managers and the requisite financial resources, costing between $50-150 per hour (Cooper, Guerin, Loftis et al., 1999, p. 100). Another complicating factor is communicating with "health care professionals who sometimes disregard your opinions because you're 'out of town'" (AARP, 1994, p.17).

Family relationships may become strained by caregiving responsibilities in any situation, and particularly for LD caregivers. Hooyman and Lustbader (1986) noted that often local siblings "resent out-of-town siblings for not doing more" (p. 51). On the other hand, LD caregiving poses "tactical and emotional challenges which are even more difficult" when there are no local family members (Hooyman & Lustbader, 1986, p. 22). Additional strains include costs of travel and long-distance calls to assess needs and arrange for care, time away from work, and emotional burdens of anxiety and guilt that caregivers may experience because they are not as available as they feel they should be.

As previously noted, little empirical research has examined LD caregiving, and most studies have focused on the "primary" or "principal" caregiver, usually a local family member. Schoonover et al. (1988) studied parent care and "geographically distant" children (living more than 50 miles away). They interviewed 100 women who were primary caregivers for elderly widowed mothers and their local siblings and sent questionnaires to distant brothers and sisters. More than half of the distant siblings reported "they sometimes felt helpless and nervous about the mother's need for help" (p. 482). While most reported no interferences in family finances or activities due to caregiving, 80% reported "at least some strain" caused by living at a distance (p. 482).

Comparing data from 1987 and 1997 national telephone surveys of caregivers, Wagner (1997b) noted "an observable increase" in the number of respondents living more than 20 minutes away from the care recipient: 16% in 1987 and 24% in 1997, and for employed caregivers,

14% in 1987 and 34% in 1997. Wagner cautioned, however, that it was not possible to determine the precise increase in long-distance caregiving, because, unlike the 1997 study, the 1987 study did not ask respondents if they lived more than an hour from the care receiver (1997b, p. 3).

The National Council on Aging (NCOA) conducted a telephone survey of 200 adults, focusing solely on LD caregiving, defined as providing or managing care, services, financial or legal assistance for a person age 55 or older who lives at least an hour away. Respondents lived, on average, 304 miles from the care recipient, requiring an average of 4 hours travel time to reach that person. The "typical" LD caregiver was a 46-year-old woman, a college graduate with a household income of $54,240, working full-time and providing assistance to her mother over a 5-year time period. The "typical" LD caregiver was a secondary caregiver, helping a primary caregiving relative who lived near the care receiver. Long distance caregivers provided services directly (52%), made arrangements for services (28%), both provided and arranged for services (19%), and paid for services (44%). Forty-one percent reported having difficulty finding care, and most (79%) reported some level of stress.

METHODOLOGY

The research method for this paper was secondary analysis of the 1997 NAC/AARP national survey of family caregivers of older adults, focused on the long-distance caregivers subgroup data. The original study was a telephone survey with a nationwide random sample of caregivers aged 18 and over. Black, Hispanic, and Asian caregivers were oversampled to ensure adequate numbers of each of these groups for analytic purposes. NAC contracted with the ICR Survey Research Group, Inc., of Media, PA, to generate the samples and conduct the survey.

Two samples were used to conduct the survey. The first was a fully replicated, stratified, single-stage random-digit-dial (RDD) sample of U.S. telephone households generated in-house by ICR. The supplemental sample was extracted from ICR's EXCEL Omnibus Service, and included individuals who had previously identified as Hispanic, Black, or Other Race. . . . In total (both samples), 1,509 telephone interviews were conducted, all in English, and averaging 20 minutes in length (NAC/AARP, 1997, p. 38).

Although the results of this study were published, no specific analysis was completed on LD caregivers, nor was the term defined. One question asked respondents to identify the amount of time between caregiver and care recipient, ranging from living in the same household to over two hours apart. Three fourths (74.9%, $n = 1130$) of respondents lived in the same household with the care recipient or within 20 minutes; 13.7% ($n = 207$) lived between 20 minutes and an hour away; 3.9% ($n = 59$) lived one to two hours away. Finally, 7.2% (n = 109) reported living more than two hours away.

Definition of the Long Distance Caregiver

As previously noted, "long-distance" caregiving has either not been defined in the literature or has been defined as the caregiver living more than 50 miles or at least an hour from the care receiver. While the NCOA study, focused specifically on long-distance caregivers, used the more-than-an hour criterion, the average travel time for that sample was 4 hours. Because the NAC/AARP data set identified caregivers living more than 2 hours away from the care receiver, we selected this as the definition for LD caregivers for this study to more closely align with the NCOA study findings and to explore characteristics and experiences of caregivers who are geographically the most distant. The purpose is of this study was to further our understanding of this specific population, by answering the following questions: Who provided LD caregiving? Who received assistance from the LD caregiver? What types of care were provided? What was the reported stress of LD caregivers? What resources/supports assisted the LD caregiver?

RESULTS

Long Distance Caregivers and Care Receivers

Table 1 summarizes demographics of the long distance (LD) caregiver. The majority were women (56%), married (65.1%), middle aged ($M = 42$ years), and half had children or grandchildren living with them. The distribution on race/ethnicity was 32.1% white, non-Hispanic; 33.9% Asian/Oriental/Chinese; 22% Hispanic, and 11.9% black. This distribution reflects the oversampling by race/ethnic group in the original study from which the LD data were drawn. Respondents reported a high level of educational attainment, with 35.8% having graduated from college, and another 16.5% reporting graduate school education. More than two-thirds were employed, and the median total annual household income fell into the $30,000-$40,000 range. The average

TABLE 1. Demographics of the Long Distance Caregiver ($\underline{N}$ = 109)

Variable	Statistic
Age	$\underline{M}$ = 42.43 years, $\underline{SD}$ = 14.54
	Range = 18-79
Gender	
Female	56%, $\underline{n}$ = 61
Male	44%, $\underline{n}$ = 48
Race	
White, non-Hispanic	32.1%, $\underline{n}$ = 35
Asian/Oriental/Chinese	33.9%, $\underline{n}$ = 37
Hispanic	22.0%, $\underline{n}$ = 24
Black	11.9%, $\underline{n}$ = 13
Marital Status	
Married	65.1%, $\underline{n}$ = 71
Single	20.2%, $\underline{n}$ = 22
Divorced/separated	11.0%, $\underline{n}$ = 12
Widowed	2.8%, $\underline{n}$ = 3
Children/grandchildren in home	
Yes	50.5%, $\underline{n}$ = 55
No	48.6%, $\underline{n}$ = 53
Education	
Less than high school graduate	6.4%, $\underline{n}$ = 7
High school graduate	17.4%, $\underline{n}$ = 19
Some college	21.1%, $\underline{n}$ = 23
Graduated college	35.8%, $\underline{n}$ = 39
Graduate school or more	16.5%, $\underline{n}$ = 18
Technical school/other	1.8%, $\underline{n}$ = 2
Refused	.9%, $\underline{n}$ = 1
Employed	
Yes	70.6%, $\underline{n}$ = 77
No	28.5%, $\underline{n}$ = 31
Total (all sources) annual household income	
Less than $10,000	5.5%, $\underline{n}$ = 6
$10,000 but less than $15,000	3.7%, $\underline{n}$ = 4
$15,000 but less than $20,000	8.3%, $\underline{n}$ = 9
$20,000 but less than $25,000	11.0%, $\underline{n}$ = 12
$25,000 but less than $30,000	9.2%, $\underline{n}$ = 10
$30,000 but less than $40,000	11.9%, $\underline{n}$ = 13
$40,000 but less than $50,000	7.3%, $\underline{n}$ = 8
$50,000 but less than $75,000	13.8%, $\underline{n}$ = 15
$75,000 and over	18.3%, $\underline{n}$ = 20
Don't know/refused	11.0%, $\underline{n}$ = 12
Length of care giving	$\underline{M}$ = 5.22, $\underline{SD}$ = 3.6
	Range = 1-30 years
Estimated hours per week providing help*	
1-3 hours	48.0%, $\underline{n}$ = 37
4-8 hours	22.1%, $\underline{n}$ = 17
10 or more hours	29.9%, $\underline{n}$ = 23

* Excludes $\underline{n}$ = 13 who reported providing "constant care" and $\underline{n}$ = 19 who reported "don't know"

length of time that care was provided was 5.22 years, and of those not providing constant care, 48% spent 1-3 hours per week in caregiving. Care recipients ranged in age from 50 to 98 with a mean age of 77.6 years (see Table 2). In terms of relationship to the caregiver, 39.4% were mothers, 13.8% were fathers, and another 13.5% were grandmothers. Over half (56%) lived with another family member or friend, and only 7.3% lived in a setting providing some assistance (e.g., assisted living, nursing home). Respondents were asked to identify "the main illness or problem of the care recipient," and almost one-fourth reported "aging" as the primary problem. Excluding the 7.3% who listed Alzheimer's as the *main* illness, another 11.9% of the remaining respondents replied "yes" when asked specifically if the care recipient suffered from Alzheimer's.

Care Networks and Types of Care Provided

Only 10.5% of respondents reported themselves as primary caregivers, while 21.1% said care responsibility was split 50-50. Over two-thirds reported someone else as primary caregiver (see Table 3). Most respondents indicated that care was provided by several people, with over 20% reporting one other person providing care and over two-thirds reporting care from two to three other caregivers. Most frequently identified additional caregivers were daughters (54.1%) and sons (48.6%). Almost two-thirds (65.1%) of LD caregivers responded that their relatives were doing their fair share in caregiving, and 68.5% reported no family conflict over caregiving.

Respondents were presented with a list of 13 tasks, 7 of which were Activities of Daily Living (ADLs) and 6 Instrumental Activities of Daily Living (IADLs) and asked if they provided this type of care (see Table 4). As might be expected, LD caregivers, in general, provided fewer ADLs than IADLs. Nevertheless, over one-third assisted with medicines and helping the care recipient getting in/out of bed or chairs. Overall, the most frequently performed tasks were IADLs, with approximately two-thirds providing transportation assistance, financial management, housework, and grocery shopping. Over half also reported making arrangements for outside services (56.9%).

Long Distance Caregiving Burdens and Benefits

Employment: As previously noted, the majority of LD caregivers worked full- or part-time (see Table 5). Of those who had been em-

TABLE 2. Demographics of the Long Distance Care Recipient (N = 109)

Variable	Statistic
Age	M = 77.61 years, SD = 10.08
	Range 50-98
Relationship to long distance care giver	
Mother	39.4%, n = 43
Father	13.8%, n = 15
Grandmother	13.8%, n = 15
Mother-in-law	9.2%, n = 10
Aunt/Uncle	7.3%, n = 8
Non-relative/friend	5.5%, n = 6
Grandfather	4.6%, n = 5
Father-in-law	3.7%, n = 4
Other relatives	2.7%, n = 3
Residence of care recipient	
With another family member/friend	56.0%, n = 61
Alone in own home	21.1%, n = 23
Apartment or retirement community	15.6%, n = 17
Assisted living	4.6%, n = 5
Nursing home	1.8%, n = 2
Boarding/group home	.9%, n = 1
Type of illness or problem condition	
Chronic	67.0%, n = 73
Short-term	15.6%, n = 17
Both	11.9%, n = 13
Don't know/refused	5.5%, n = 6
Main illness or problem of care recipient	
Aging	22.0%, n = 24
Heart disease/condition	13.8%, n = 15
Diabetes	8.3%, n = 9
Alzheimer's/confusion/dementia/forgetfulness	7.3%, n = 8
Blindness/vision loss	6.4%, n = 7
Arthritis	5.5%, n = 6
Stroke	5.5%, n = 6
Mobility/can't get around	4.6%, n = 5
Don't know/refused	5.5%, n = 6
Other*	16.2%, n = 18
Does care recipient have Alzheimer's?	
Yes	11.0%, n = 12
No	81.7%, n = 89
Were not asked**	7.3%, n = 8

* All other responses where n< 5 (e.g., cancer, kidney disease, mental illness, injuries)
** Respondents who indicated Alzheimer's as main illness were not asked this specific question.

TABLE 3. Care Providers and Care Network (N = 109)

Variable	Statistic
Who provides the primary care?	
Long distance respondent	10.5%, n = 10
Someone else	68.4%, n = 65
We split it 50-50	21.1%, n = 20
How many others provide care?	
No one else provides care	12.8%, n = 14
One other person provides care	20.2%, n = 22
Two other persons provide care	34.9%, n = 38
Three other persons provide care*	32.1%, n = 35
Who provides additional care?	
Daughters	54.1%, n = 59
Son	48.6%, n = 53
Non-Relative/friend/companion	12.9%, n = 14
Spouse	9.2%, n = 10
Daughter-in-law	9.2%, n = 10
Son-in-law	9.2%, n = 10
Granddaughter	8.4%, n = 9
Niece	7.4%, n = 8
Sister	5.5%, n = 6
Grandson	5.5%, n = 6
Other relative	4.6%, n = 5
Everyone/whole family/all	3.6%, n = 4
Brother	2.7%, n = 3
Mother	1.8%, n = 2
Nephew	1.8%, n = 2
Sister-in-law	.9%, n = 1
Live-in nurses or aides (paid help)	.9%, n = 1
Volunteer	.9%, n = 1
Do other relatives who provide care do their fair share?	
Yes	65.1%, n = 71
No	18.3%, n = 20
Don't have other relatives/refused**	15.6%, n = 17
Don't know	.9%, n = 1
Extent of family conflict over caregiving*	
None at all	68.5%, n = 63
Some conflict	28.3%, n = 26
A lot of conflict	2.2%, n = 2
Don't know	1.1%, n = 1

*Respondents could only list up to three persons also providing care
** "Don't have other relatives" and "refused" were coded together in original data set
***Does not include respondents reporting no other relatives

TABLE 4. Proportion of Long Distance Caregivers Providing Type of Care (N = 109)

Variable	% Yes*
Activities of Daily Living (ADLs)*	
Giving medicines, pills, or injections	37.6%, n = 41
Get in and out of beds and chairs	36.7%, n = 40
Get dressed	29.4%, n = 32
Get to and from the toilet	25.7%, n = 28
Feeding him or her	24.8%, n = 27
Bathe or shower	22.0%, n = 24
With continence, or dealing with diapers	11.9%, n = 13
Instrumental Activities of Daily Living (IADLs)*	
Transportation	67.9%, n = 74
Managing finances	66.1%, n = 72
Housework	64.2%, n = 70
Grocery shopping	63.3%, n = 69
Preparing meals	56.9%, n = 62
Arranging/supervising outside services	56.9%, n = 62

*Respondents were asked to indicate from a list of tasks if they provided this type of care

ployed while caregiving, 61.4% reported at least one negative impact on employment. Relatively few made major changes, such as giving up work entirely or moving from full- to part-time work. In contrast, 43.2% reported they came in late, left early or took time off, and over one-third said they had taken a leave of absence, with most indicating their employers were very understanding.

Social, Physical, Emotional, and Financial Stress: Over half of LD caregivers reported they had given up vacations, hobbies, or other leisure activities, and nearly one-third indicated they had less time for other family members (see Table 5). Only 10% reported physical or mental problems resulting from their caregiving roles. LD caregivers reported greater emotional stress than physical strain, and relatively little financial hardship. One-third spent none of their own money on groceries, medicines, or other care receiver needs, and less than 3% had received public funds for care provision.

When asked what had been their biggest difficulty as a caregiver, a quarter reported none (see Table 6). The most frequently cited difficulties related to the distance from the care receiver, followed by the

TABLE 5. Employment, Social, Physical, Emotional and Financial Impacts of Long Distance Caregiving ($\underline{N}$ = 109)

Variable	Statistic
Employment Status While Providing Care	
Working full-time	54.1%, $\underline{n}$ = 59
Working part-time	16.5%, $\underline{n}$ = 18
Retired/not employed*	28.5%, $\underline{n}$ = 31
Impact of Caregiving on Employment**	
Arrived late/left early or took time off	43.2%, $\underline{n}$ = 38
Took a leave of absence	34.1%, $\underline{n}$ = 30
Gave up work entirely	8.0%, $\underline{n}$ = 7
Changed from full to part time or fewer demands	6.8%, $\underline{n}$ = 6
Turned down a promotion	5.7%, $\underline{n}$ = 5
Chose early retirement	4.5%, $\underline{n}$ = 4
Lost job benefits	3.4%, $\underline{n}$ = 3
Attitude of Employer Towards Caregiving Demands**	
Very understanding	64.8%, $\underline{n}$ = 35
Somewhat understanding	14.8%, $\underline{n}$ = 8
Not very understanding	7.4%, $\underline{n}$ = 4
Employer not aware of demands	7.4%, $\underline{n}$ = 4
Don't know	5.6%, $\underline{n}$ = 3
Social Impact (% = Yes)	
Gave up vacations, hobbies, or other activities	51.4%, $\underline{n}$ = 56
Less time for other family members	31.2%, $\underline{n}$ = 34
Suffered physical or mental problems (% = Yes)	10.1%, $\underline{n}$ = 11
Physical strain (1 = none; 5 = very much)	M = 2.05, SD = 1.55
	Range 1.75-2.34
Emotional stress (1 = none; 5 = very stressful)	M = 2.45, SD = 1.54
	Range = 2.16-2.74
Financial hardship (1 = none; 5 = great deal)	M = 1.72, SD = 1.33
	Range = 1.47-1.98
Received money from government for care (% = yes)	2.8%, $\underline{n}$ = 3
Estimated monthly amount spent for care**	
$0	33.0%, $\underline{n}$ = 34
$1-$50	14.6%, $\underline{n}$ = 15
$100-$200	27.2%, $\underline{n}$ = 28
$250-$500	17.5%, $\underline{n}$ = 18
$600-$1,000	6.8%, $\underline{n}$ = 7
$5200	.9%, $\underline{n}$ = 1

* Eleven of those not working reported having been employed at some time while providing care
**Does not include 21 respondents who never worked while providing care
***Includes only respondents who reported one or more Impacts on Employment
****Categories were developed from specific dollar amounts reported by respondents
   (e.g., no respondents reported a value between $51-99)

TABLE 6. Biggest Difficulty and Greatest Reward from Long Distance Caregiving ($\underline{N}$ = 109)

Variable	Statistic
Biggest Difficulty in Providing Care	
None	25.7%, n = 28
Inconvenient distance/location	20.2%, n = 22
Watching deterioration (emotional straining)	13.8%, n = 15
Demands on time/unable to do as want	11.0%, n = 12
Making sure s/he cared for/peace of mind	7.3%, n = 8
Communication is difficult	4.6%, n = 5
Care recipient attitude/uncooperative	3.7%, n = 4
Financial strain	3.7%, n = 4
Difficulties with physical demands	3.7%, n = 4
Weight of decision making	1.8%, n = 2
Not enough help from others	1.8%, n = 2
Don't know/other	1.8%, n = 2
Dealing with family members	.9%, n = 1
Greatest Reward from Providing Long Distance Care	
Personal satisfaction/doing a good deed	19.3%, n = 21
Family loyalty/giving back/obligation	18.3%, n = 20
Appreciation/happiness of care receiver	18.3%, n = 20
Knowing recipient is well cared for	10.2%, n = 11
Sharing his/her time; spending time together	10.1%, n = 11
Watching health improve	9.2%, n = 10
None/no greatest reward	5.5%, n = 6
Love, nice to me, care, we're friends	4.6%, n = 5
Source of family strength	1.8%, n = 2
Religious reasons	.9%, n = 1
Someone will do same for me	.9%, n = 1
Don't know	.9%, n = 1

emotional strain of watching the deterioration of their loved one. Respondents also identified caregiving rewards; the most frequently cited were personal satisfaction from doing a good deed, family loyalty and a sense of "giving back," and appreciation from the care receiver.

Services and Supports

LD caregivers were asked about types of services they had used in caregiving, and 98 responded to a series of questions about services (see Table 7). The most frequently used services were assistive devices, such as wheelchairs and walkers, followed by home modification, and personal or nursing care service. The primary reason identified for non-use of all services was "no need." However, the second reason identified varied by type of service. For example, 15 respondents did not use support groups because they were too busy. For adult day care, 10 respondents indicated the care recipient or caregiver was too proud to accept the service. Respondents reported being unaware of some services (e.g., support groups, financial information), but few reported services not available to them (e.g., temporary care, adult day care).

DISCUSSION

The findings of this study provide a snapshot of a small sample of LD caregivers–their characteristics, perceptions about their caregiving role, and service pattern usage. While it was not the purpose of the study to compare LD caregivers to other caregivers in the NAC/AARP sample, the findings do, in fact, indicate some differences that were also found in the NCOA study of 200 LD caregivers. Comparisons between the LD caregivers in the NAC/AARP and NCOA samples must be interpreted with caution. Although both were telephone surveys, the NAC/AARP sample was drawn to obtain overrepresentation of racial/ethnic populations; the NCOA study used an omnibus survey panel of respondents representative of the U.S. adult population. The surveys included different questions; similar questions were worded in ways that did not allow for comparison. Additionally, "long distance" was defined differently in these studies.

With these caveats in mind, some similarities and differences seemed to emerge. While 73% of all caregivers in the NAC/AARP study were women, only 56% of the LD caregivers were women; similarly, in the NCOA study, 54% of LD caregivers were women. LD caregivers reported higher educational attainment and income than other caregivers. For example, 52% of LD caregivers in the NAC/AARP study had earned a college degree or had done graduate study, compared to 29% of all caregivers in that sample. In the NCOA study, 48% of LD caregivers reported having a college degree or graduate education, com-

TABLE 7. Services and Supports Used by Long Distance Caregivers ($\underline{N}$ = 98*)

Variable	Statistic	
	Used service	No Need for service**
Assistive device	38.8%, n = 38	94.9%, n = 56
Home modification	34.5%, n = 30	92.7%, n = 51
Personal/Nursing	25.5%, n = 25	80.8%, n = 59
Financial information	20.4%, n = 20	71.8%, n = 56
Housework	19.4%, n = 19	87.2%, n = 68
Transportation	17.3%, n = 17	92.6%, n = 75
Meal service	15.3%, n = 15	90.2%, n = 74
Temporary/Respite Care Service	12.2%, n = 12	70.6%, n = 60
Adult Day Care/Senior Center	12.2%, n=12	64.3%, n = 54
Support groups	7.1%, n = 7	49.5%, n = 45

* Percentage excludes 11 of the 109 respondents who replied "don't know" or "refused" for all
  services and supports
**Proportion of those who did not use service/support because of no need

pared to 30% in the NCOA's omnibus survey panel of 10,000 respondents from which the 200 LD caregivers were identified. These findings align with observations by Schoonover et al. (1988) that upwardly mobile adult children and those of higher social status are more likely to live at a distance from parents.

LD caregivers in the NAC/AARP and the NCOA studies reported other similarities: the average length of caregiving was approximately 5 years (4.5 years average for all NAC/AARP caregivers); 50% of the NAC/AARP and 57% of NCOA respondents had been caregiving for 3 years or less. The NAC/AARP and NCOA/LD caregivers were comparable in the estimated time involved in caregiving; approximately 30% of the NAC/AARP and 25% of NCOA/LD caregivers spent 10 or more hours per week, and the remaining LD caregivers in both studies spent fewer hours per week in caregiving. In the NAC/AARP study, *all* caregivers provided care on average 17.9 hours per week, a difference that may be attributed to the fact that one-fifth of care recipients lived in the same household as the caregiver or were in closer proximity. Given the two hour distance, it is not surprising that a higher proportion of LD caregivers would provide IADL's in contrast to ADL's; this pattern held true for LD caregivers in the NCOA study, and the total sample of caregivers in the NAC/AARP study. Over one-fourth of the LD care-givers in the current study provided care in five of the seven ADL cate-gories, but we do not know how frequently tasks were performed, on a regular basis during weekly or monthly visits, or occasionally in provid-ing "respite" to local caregivers.

Living arrangements of care receivers differed substantially. Only 7.5% of LD care receivers in the NAC/AARP study resided in nursing homes or group settings in contrast to 26% of NCOA study care. This difference might reflect disparities in health status of care receivers in these two studies, which would likely affect care demands and impacts on LD caregivers. Wagner (1997a) pointed out, however, that nursing home placement does not necessarily end the family member's caregiving role: "Many caregivers continue to take an active role in care management and advocacy on behalf of the elder and continue to see themselves as 'caregivers'" (p. 14).

In both studies of LD caregivers, a higher percentage than might be expected reported themselves as assuming or sharing primary caregiver responsibilities. In the current study, nearly 11% reported themselves as providing primary care, while another 21% shared primary care 50/50 with someone else. In the NCOA study, 21% reported themselves as the primary caregiver, with an additional 31% reporting equally shared re-sponsibility. Thus, between one-third and one-half of LD caregivers are *not* secondary helpers, as might be assumed given the distance between them and the care receiver. Health and human service professionals working with frail, older populations must consider LD caregivers as an important part of the care network and not discount them. The roles they play as primary caregivers and the contributions they make in support-ing local caregivers are critical for meeting care recipient needs. Per-haps explicating and legitimizing the role of LD caregivers might normalize this experience and reduce guilt related to not being physi-cally accessible to the care receiver.

As a secondary data analysis, the primary limitations of this study are related to the methodology of the original NAC/AARP study. Because it was a telephone survey, it excluded those without telephones and, therefore, possibly the poorest U.S. residents. In addition, while sam-pling was done to ensure adequate numbers of minority populations for purposes of data analysis, respondents who did not speak English were excluded. The data reflect only perceptions of caregivers and not care receivers or others in the support network. Additionally, this secondary analysis was limited to the questions asked in the original study, which may not have captured all the distinctive experiences and needs of LD caregivers. Finally, the total of only 109 LD caregiving respondents limited multivariate analysis for groups within the sample, particularly racial and ethnic groups.

Additional research is needed in light of the anticipated growth of LD caregivers and limited generalizability of current study findings. The definition of "long distance" needs to be carefully considered, because both time and distance are relative concepts and previous studies have used different definitions. Additionally, race, ethnicity, and income differences among LD caregivers need further exploration to identify culturally relevant services that are accessible, particularly for individuals with limited incomes.

REFERENCES

American Association of Retired Persons. (1994) *Miles away and still caring: A guide for long-distance caregivers.* Washington, DC: AARP.

Barer, B. M., & Johnson, C.L. (1990). A critique of the caregiving literature. *The Gerontologist, 30* (1), 26-29.

Biegel, D.E. (1995). Caregiver burden. In G.K. Maddox (Ed.), *The Encyclopedia of Aging: A Comprehensive Resource in Gerontology and Geriatrics* (pp. 138-141). New York: Springer.

Brody, E.M. (1985). Parent care as a normative family stress. The Gerontologist, *25* (1), 19-29.

Cantor, M.H. (1983). Strain among caregivers: A study of experience in the United States. *The Gerontologist, 23* (6), 597-604.

Carton, E. (2000). Long distance caring. *Caregiver.Com. Today's Caregiver Magazine. www.caregiver.com*

Cooper, J.H., Guerin, J.F., Loftis, J.B., et al. (1999). *Fourteen friends' guide to eldercaring: Practical advice, inspiration, shared experiences, space for your thoughts.* Sterling, VA: Capital Books.

George, L.K., & Gwyther, L.P. (1986). Caregiver well-being: A multidimensional examination of family caregivers of demented adults. *The Gerontologist, 26* (3), 253-259.

Heath, A. (1993). *Long distance caregiving: A survival guide for far away caregivers.* Lakewood, CO: American Source Books.

Hooyman, N.R., & Lustbader, W. (1986). Taking care of your aging family members: A practical guide. New York: Free Press/Macmillan.

Montgomery, R.J.V., Gonyea, J.G., & Hooyman, N.R. (1985). Caregiving and the experience of subjective and objective burden. *Family Relations, 34*(1), 19-26.

Mui, A.C. (1995). Caring for frail elderly parents: A comparison of adult sons and daughters. *The Gerontologist, 35* (1), 86-93.

National Alliance for Caregiving and The American Association of Retired Persons (1997). *Family caregiving in the U.S. Findings from a national survey.* Bethesda, MD: NAC & Washington, DC: AARP.

National Council on Aging. www.ncoa.org.

National Family Caregivers Association. (2000). *A national report on the status of caregiving in America.* Kensington, MD: NCFA.

Pearlin, L.I., Mullan, J.T., Semple, S.J., and Skaff, M.M. (1990). Caregiving and the stress process: An overview of concepts and their measures. *The Gerontologist, 30* (5), 583-594.

Penrod, J.D., Kane, R.A., Kane, R.L., & Finch, M.D. (1995). Who cares? The size, scope, and composition of the caregiver support system. *The Gerontologist, 35*(4), 489-497.

Schoonover, C.B., Brody, E.M., Hoffman, C., & Kleban, M.H. (1988). Parent care and geographically distant children. *Research on Aging, 10* (4), 472-492.

Stone, R., Cafferata, G.L., Sangl, J. (1987). Caregivers of the frail elderly: A national profile. *The Gerontologist, 27* (5), 616-626.

Toseland, R.W., & Rossiter, C.M. (1996). Social work practice with family caregivers of frail older persons. In M.J. Holosko & M.D. Feit (Eds.), *Social Work Practice with the Elderly, Second Edition* (pp.299-320). Toronto, Canadian Scholars Press.

Wagner, D. L. (1997a). *Caring across the miles: Findings of a survey of long-distance caregivers.* Washington, DC: NCOA.

Wagner, D.L. (1997b). *Comparative analysis of caregiver data for caregivers to the elderly 1987 and 1997.* Bethesda, MD: National Alliance for Caregiving.

Weaver, T. (2001). Caring for an elder from far away: Geriatric care managers. *Caregiver.Com: Today's Caregiver Magazine.* www.caregiver.com.

Zarit, S.H., Reever, K.E., & Bach-Peterson, J. (1980). Relatives of the impaired elderly: Correlates of feelings of burden. *The Gerontologist, 20* (6), 649-655.

Elder Abuse Intervention Strategies: Social Service or Criminal Justice?

Patricia Brownell, CSW, PhD
Agata Wolden, MSW

SUMMARY. The debate in the field of elder abuse as to whether elder abuse is caused by caregiver stress or abuser impairment has precipitated a discussion as to whether elder abuse should be considered a social service issue, or a criminal justice problem (Wolf, 1999). Even when family violence rises to the level of a crime as defined by state penal code, some professionals argue that a social service approach is best suited to address this social problem. The study presented here compares an elder abuse program providing social

Patricia Brownell is Assistant Professor at the Fordham University Graduate School of Social Service. She is a John A. Hartford Geriatric Social Work Faculty Scholar, and her research focuses on elder abuse and neglect. Prior to joining the Fordham faculty in 1995, Dr. Brownell served 26 years in the Human Resources Administration, the social services arm of the municipal government in New York City. Agata Wolden graduated from the Fordham University Graduate School of Social Service in 2002. She served her field placement at Walk the Walk as a research and clinical intern. She collected and analyzed data for the study at Walk the Walk with a stipend from the John A. Hartford Foundation. Ms. Wolden was a lawyer in Poland, her native country, and is currently a social worker at Wyckhoff Heights Hospital, Brooklyn, NY.

[Haworth co-indexing entry note]: "Elder Abuse Intervention Strategies: Social Service or Criminal Justice?" Brownell, Patricia, and Agata Wolden. Co-published simultaneously in *Journal of Gerontological Social Work* (The Haworth Social Work Practice Press, an imprint of The Haworth Press, Inc.) Vol. 40, No. 1/2, 2002, pp. 83-100; and: *Older People and Their Caregivers Across the Spectrum of Care* (ed: Judith L. Howe) The Haworth Social Work Practice Press, an imprint of The Haworth Press, Inc., 2003, pp. 83-100. Single or multiple copies of this article are available for a fee from The Haworth Document Delivery Service [1-800-HAWORTH, 9:00 a.m. - 5:00 p.m. (EST). E-mail address: docdelivery@haworthpress.com].

10.1300/J083v40n01_06

services to elder abuse victims with another serving elderly victims of crimes. *[Article copies available for a fee from The Haworth Document Delivery Service: 1-800-HAWORTH. E-mail address: <docdelivery@haworthpress.com> Website: <http://www.HaworthPress.com> © 2002 by The Haworth Press, Inc. All rights reserved.]*

KEYWORDS. Elder abuse and neglect, gerontological social work, social services, criminal justice, elder abuse service delivery, aging, interdisciplinary, community based services, domestic violence, elder abuse interventions

INTRODUCTION

Service interventions evolve from theories about causes of social problems. Two current theories of elder abuse etiology are those of *caregiver stress* and *abuser impairment* (Pillemer & Finkelhor, 1989; Steinmetz, 1980). The definition of abuser impairment has been further expanded to include abuser criminality (Brownell, Berman, & Salamone, 1999).

While domestic violence or abuse of an older adult aged 60 years and above by an intimate represents one subset of elder abuse, stranger crime against older adults has also been identified as a form of elder abuse (Yin, 1984). Both domestic violence and stranger crime may involve criminal acts as well as actions that, while harmful and hurtful to the victim, do not rise to the level of a crime as defined by state penal codes. For the purpose of this discussion, abuser impairment may include health, mental health, emotional, and substance abuse disorders.

Caregiver Stress

Early studies of elder abuse and neglect examined characteristics of the victim as predictors of elder abuse, and suggested that frail health and dependency on the part of the elderly victims caused caregivers to experience such a high level of stress that they became abusive. This explanatory theory was proposed by sociologist Suzanne Steinmetz to explain why elder abuse occurs (Steinmetz, 1980). The typical profile of the elder abuse victim and perpetrator as described by early elder abuse studies was that of a spouse or adult child, typically a daughter, who abused and neglected their care dependent family member because they were overwhelmed by the demands of caregiving.

Abuser Impairment

Later studies examined the characteristics of the abusers as predictive of elder abuse (Pillemer & Finkelhor, 1989). The findings of these studies suggested that abuser impairment, such as untreated mental illness, substance abuse, dementia, and socio-pathology, explained elder abuse and neglect of elderly family members, who may be primary supports or caregivers of their abusers. Proponents of this theoretical perspective described a typical profile of elder abuse as involving an impaired spouse or adult child perpetrator who abuses an elderly family member to assert power, to obtain resources by coercion, or because an impairment distorts his or her ability to control violent behavior or to exercise sound judgment.

Implications for Service Interventions

The debate in the field of elder abuse as to whether elder abuse is caused by caregiver stress or abuser impairment has precipitated a discussion as to whether elder abuse should be considered a social service issue, or a criminal justice problem (Wolf, 1999). Even when family violence rises to the level of a crime as defined by state penal code, some professionals argue that a family service approach is best suited to address this social problem.

Proponents of the criminal justice response argue that like child and spouse/partner abuse, perpetrators, even if impaired, must be held accountable for their acts (Brandl, 2000). From this perspective, a legal response–including the courts, law enforcement, district attorney and penal system–is most effective in addressing the problem of elder abuse and neglect.

According to Bergeron (2001), theories held by practitioners inform practice, guide case assessment processes, and shape interventions. Depending on how an elder abuse case situation comes to the attention of the program and the theoretical perspective underlying that program, it may be treated as a social service or a legal/criminal justice problem. However, to date little is known about the distinctions between profiles of elder abuse situations that become defined as social service or criminal justice problems, including the abusive actions that precipitate professional involvement; the services that constitute social service or criminal justice intervention; and the outcomes of these interventions, particularly whether or not they are deemed successful in addressing the abuse situation.

A number of questions remain unanswered regarding how elder abuse cases come to be identified as a social service or a legal problem. What elder abuse situations come to the attention of social service as opposed to crime victim programs? What is the demographic profile of victims and abusers including gender, race/ethnicity, and relationship between victim and abuser? What are the services provided by social service programs in contrast to legal or criminal justice programs? What are the service outcomes for each type of intervention: how are they different and how are the similar?

To address these questions, a research project was undertaken by the Fordham University Graduate School of Social Service, in collaboration with Walk the Walk, Inc., with funding from the John A. Hartford Foundation. The data were collected and analyzed by a Hartford Social Work Research intern, under the direction of a Hartford Geriatric Social Work Faculty Scholar.

DATA AND METHODOLOGY

Walk the Walk, Inc. is a community based organization located in Queens, New York serving elder abuse victims and their families. Walk the Walk operates a substance and alcohol abuse program (Alpha/Omega), a legal referral and information program (Elder Law Institute) and a community based case management program (STEPS–Services to Empower Seniors). Another program component, Mary's House, the first full-service elder abuse shelter in the country, is in the process of completion.

The study examines two community based elder abuse case management programs operated under the STEPS umbrella: (1) the Crime Victims Board (CVB) program, funded by the New York State Crime Victims Board, and (2) the Department for the Aging (DFTA) Elder Services (ES) Program, a social service program funded by the New York City Department for the Aging. While both programs are funded to serve elder abuse victims and their families, the CVB program focuses on providing legal services to victims of crimes or alleged crimes, and the ES program provides social services to elder abuse victims and their families when the abuse does not appear to have risen to the level of a crime as defined by the New York State Penal Code.

Hypotheses Tested

Two hypotheses were formulated and tested. The first hypothesis was that for cases where the abuse or neglect is defined as a crime by the New York State Penal Code, a criminal justice intervention is more effective than a social service intervention in achieving the desired outcome of client safety.

The second hypothesis is that for cases in which the abuse or neglect is not defined as a crime by the New York State Penal Code, a social service intervention is more effective than a criminal justice intervention in achieving the desired outcome of client safety.

The desired outcome of client safety is further operationalized as the successful implementation of the service plan achieved (resolution) at the point in time that the case was closed. This operational definition has been used in other elder abuse program evaluations to evaluate intervention outcomes (Wolf & Pillemer, 2000).

Additional Research Questions

Additional research questions formulated from the Research Agenda on Abuse of Older Persons and Adults with Disabilities (Wolf, 1998) include:

- Are there differences in client/perpetrator demographic and abuse profiles between the Crime Victims and Family Services Program caseloads?
- Are there differences in referral sources?
- Are there differences in services delivered?
- Are there differences in client safety outcomes between the Crime Victims and Family Service Programs?
- Are there differences in client safety outcomes related to type of abuse?

Study Design

A non-experimental study design was used to compare elder abuse situations served by the Walk the Walk STEPS' Crime Victims Program with those served by the STEPS' Elder Services Program. This included socio-demographic profiles of the victims and abusers, types and circumstances of abuse, service interventions, and service outcomes. Walk the Walk has been in operation since 1997. Only closed cases were examined as part of the study, to make possible a comparison of service outcomes. There were approximately 700 closed cases since the STEPS program became operational, with a current active caseload of 300. Because of the large number of closed cases, a decision was made to draw a random sample of cases from those cases closed in 2001. A random sample of 30 cases out of approximately 69 Elder Services (ES) cases and 30 cases out of 78 CVB cases was selected from closed files, for a total of 60 cases. There were four cases among the sample where the victim had died of causes unrelated to abuse or neglect. These cases were not analyzed as part of the study, bringing the total number of cases analyzed to 56: 27 from the Elder Services Program, and 29 from the Crime Victims Program.

The case records included an intake application, which provided demographic information about the victim and when available about the abuser, victims' living arrangements, referral sources, abuse situation description, needs assessment and service plan, interventions provided, and service outcomes. Cases were closed when service goals were met, or when the victim terminated, disappeared, no longer needed services, or died.

To ensure confidentiality of the victims' identity, names, social security numbers, and addresses were concealed prior to review by the researcher. A data collection form was created to transpose case information from the case records for data entry purposes. Cases were selected based on the following criteria: the victim was 60 years of age and older; the victim experienced physical, financial, or psychological, or neglect, including self-neglect; and the case had been closed so a service outcome could be determined. Data collection took place during the Spring 2002.

Variables, Measurements, and Operations

Socio-demographic variables of victims, and when available perpetrators, included age, gender, marital status, and race/ethnicity. Variables related to victim and when available perpetrator living arrangements included borough of resident, living alone, with others, and with perpetrator. Variables related to victims' health, mental health and cognitive status, and when available that of perpetrators as well, were coded as nominal variables. A variable pertaining to personal problems was added to include situations related to divorce, separation from partner, or related family disruptions. Relationships between victim and perpetrator were coded as child, grandchild, spouse, partner, friend/neighbor, other relatives, non-relatives (including strangers), and self. Referral sources were also included as variables in the study.

Abuse situations that met the definition of a criminal act as defined by the New York State Penal Code included: assault, menacing, burglary, larceny, extortion, physical abuse, sexual abuse, forgery, robbery, stalking, and harassment, which could be verbal or financial. Abuse situations that reflected social problems included eviction (reflecting self-neglect), neglect, abandonment, social confinement, and needs for social entitlements and other personal social services. Outcomes related to the implementation of the service plans that addressed the abuse situation included: safety achieved through successful implementation of the service plan; safety achieved unrelated to implementation of the service plan; and safety not achieved. The latter category included case situations where the victim terminated services or disappeared before safety was achieved through implementation of the service plan.

Analytic Strategy

Univariate and bivariate statistics were used to describe the profile of victims who were served in the programs, the victims' abusers and the abuse situations that brought them to the attention of Walk the Walk. For purposes of the analysis, race/ethnic categories were coded as minority/non-minority. Victim Health problems were recoded as: physical health, mental health, cognitive impairment, and alcohol/drug (substance) abuse. Living arrangements were recoded as: lives alone, lives with others, and lives with perpetrator alone, and lives with perpetrator and others. Source of referrals were coded as: self, relatives, social service agency, police, home care agency, hospital, and other. Relationship with perpetrator included: child, grandchild, spouse, partner (including intimate partner), friend/neighbor, other non-relative, and no perpetrator for the self-neglect cases. Perpetrator problems were recoded as: alcohol/drugs (substance abuse), financial, mental health, legal, and personal. Personal problems included divorce, separation and other relationship problems. Abuse, whether or not it rose to the level of a criminal act, was recategorized as physical, financial, and psychological.

Service interventions were recategorized as legal intervention if they included contact with law enforcement; criminal or family court action, for example, for an order of protection, consultation with legal services; or involvement with District Attorneys, offices. Service interventions were recategorized as social service interventions if they included counseling, linkage with health or mental health services, delivery of home care or entitlement services, or help with evictions.

A t-test was used to determine if the ages of Elder Service Program clients differed significantly from the ages of Crime Victims Program clients. Chi-square tests of association were utilized to determine if the hypotheses posed by the study were supported by the data. Chi-square tests of association are used with nominal or categorical variables to assess the extent to which observed frequencies differ from what would be expected by chance alone (Rubin & Babbie, 2001).

FINDINGS

Description of Sample

Gender: The majority of victims served by the two programs were female: 43 (76.8%), as compared with 13 (23.2%) male. The gender breakdown for both programs was similar. The Elder Service Program served 20 (74.1%) women as compared with the Crime Victims Program (23 or 79.3% female).

Age: The average age of the 55 victims for whom exact age could be determined was 77.4, with a standard deviation of 7.54. The youngest victim was age 60 and the oldest victim was age 94. There was no statistical difference in the average age of victims served by either the Crime Victims or Elder Service Programs. There was no difference in the ages of female and male victims in either program.

Race/Ethnicity: The majority of victims were White or non-minority (33 or 60%) as opposed to minority (Black, Asian, American Indian, or Pacific Islander, or Hispanic–a linguistic category) during the time period covered by the study. There were a total of 22 (40%) minority victims in both programs. However there were slightly more minority victims served by the Crime Victims Program than the Family Service Program (13 as compared to 9). Proportionately, there were more non-minority clients served by the Elder Service Program (17 or 65.4%), compared with 9 or 34.6% minority. The Crime victims program served an almost equal number of minority and non-minority victims (13 or 54.8% minority as compared with 15 or 55.2% non-minority).

Marital Status: The majority of victims (50 or almost 90%) were not married, with 6 (10.7%) married. Of the unmarried victims, 24 (42.9%) were single or divorced, and 26 (46.4%) were widowed. In the Crime Victims Program, the largest category of clients was that of widowed (9 or

31%), while in the Elder Service Program, the largest category of clients was that of single or divorced (15 or 55%).

Health Status: A total of 48 case records included information about victims' health and mental health status. Of these, 30 reported some level of physical impairment, and the majority of these victims were receiving services from the Elder Service Program (17 or 68%, as compared with 13 or 56% physically impaired victims served by the Crime Victims Program. Eleven victims were identified as having mental health problems, and an additional 10 victims were identified with cognitive impairments. Only one victim was identified as having problems with substance abuse (alcohol). Impaired victims, by category, were fairly evenly divided between the Elder Service and Crime Victims Programs, with the one substance abusing victim served by the Crime Victims Program.

Living Arrangements: The largest group of victims lived with their abusers (22 or 40%), with an additional 6 reported as living with their abusers and others. The second largest group of victims lived alone (21 or 38.2%). Six victims lived with others but not their abusers. The largest category of victims served by the Family Service Program lived alone (14 or 51.9%, as compared with 7 or 25% of victims served by the Crime Victims Program). The largest category of victims served by the Crime Victims Program lived with their abusers (14 or 50%), compared with this category of victim served by the Elder Service Program (8 or 29.6%).

Referral Sources: Referrals for Walk the Walk STEPS services were made by victims' family members, usually adult children (16 or 28.6%); victim self-referral (12 victims or 21.4% self-reported victimization); social service agency (12 or 21.4 victims); hospital social workers (4 or 7.1%); home care agencies, specifically the Visiting Nurse Service (4 or 7.1%); and the police (3 or 5.4%). An additional 2 victims were referred from other sources. These include one victim referred by a bank manager and another referred by a building superintendent. Family members were the most likely to make referrals to the Crime Victims Program (10 or 34.5%), and victims themselves were the most likely to self-refer to the Elder Service Program (7 or 25.9%).

Relationships Between Perpetrators and Victims: Perpetrators were most likely to be adult children of victims (18 or 32%). The next most likely category of abuse was self-neglect: 9 or 16.1% of abuse situations did not include a perpetrator. However, differences emerged in the profile of cases served by the Crime Victims as compared with the Elder Service Program. Victims served by the Crime Victims Program were twice as likely as those served by the Elder Service Program to be victimized by their adult children (12 or 41.4% of Crime Victims Program cases, as compared with 6 or 22.2% of Family Service Program cases). Victims of grandchildren were equally likely to be served by Crime Victims as the Elder Service Program (3 or 10.3% as compared with 3 or 11.1%). As might be expected, all the self-neglect cases were served by the Family Service Program (9 or 33.3% of the Elder Service Program caseload sample). Spouse abuse was the smallest category of abuser-victim cases in the sample, with the Crime Victims Program and the Elder Service Program serving one spouse abuse case each.

Perpetrator Characteristics: Data on perpetrators were limited by lack of information in the case records. However, 20 or 35.7% included the perpetrators' ages, and 27 or 48% of cases included information on perpetrator characteristics pertaining to identified problem or problems. The average age among this group of perpetrators was 41 years, with the youngest 16 years and the oldest 86 years. Twenty-seven (27) perpetrators were identified as having a total of 36 problems. The most common were problems with substance abuse (drugs and alcohol), and financial problems. A total of 14 perpetrators were identified as having substance abuse problems and 14 were identified as having financial problems. One perpetrator was identified with mental health problems, and one with legal problems. Six perpetrators were identified as having personal problems, defined as divorce, separation or other intimate partnership difficulties.

Description of Program Interventions

Legal Interventions: Of the 56 cases randomly selected for analysis, 17 or 30% involved legal interventions. Of these, 13 were CVB cases and 4 were FS cases. Legal interventions undertaken by the FS Program did not involve the criminal justice system. Rather, they related to eviction proceedings in housing court. Legal interventions undertaken by the CVB Program included applying for orders of protection in family or criminal courts, engaging law enforcement, and working with the District Attorneys' offices to prosecute an abuser.

Social Service Interventions: A total of 49 cases involved social service interventions. Of these, 25 cases were served by the ES Program and 24 cases were served by the CVB Program. Social services included counseling, referrals, and linkages to health and mental health services, assistance in obtaining entitlements and other in-home and community-based services for older adults, and housing assistance other than legal services related to housing court proceedings. The almost even distribution of social service interventions across both programs suggests the importance of social service provision in elder abuse situations where the abuse rises to the level of a crime, as well as in elder abuse cases where the abuse does not rise to the level of a crime.

Types of Abuse Addressed by Elder Abuse Programs

Financial Abuse: A total of 27 cases involved financial abuse. Of these, 6 were served by the ES Program and 21 were served by the CVB Program.

Psychological Abuse: Of the 14 cases with reported psychological abuse, 3 were served by the ES Program and 11 were served by the CVB Program.

Physical Abuse: A total of 14 cases included reports of physical abuse. Of these, 3 were served by the ES Program and 11 were served by the CVB Program.

Neglect: Of the 7 cases with reported neglect, 3 were served by the ES Program and 4 were served by the CVB Program.

Social Problems: A total of 23 cases included reported social problems. Of these, 15 were served by the ES Program and 8 were served by the CVB Program. In the 8 cases served by the CVB Program, the identified social problems were secondary to the criminal abuse situations presented as primary problems.

OUTCOMES FOR FS AND CVB ELDER ABUSE CASES

Resolved and Unresolved Cases

Resolved Cases: For a case to be successfully resolved at the time of case closing, the objective of client safety had to be met. Resolution, or the objective of victim safety, could be achieved in one of two ways. The first is the achievement of victim safety through the successful implementation of the intervention plan. The second is the achievement of victim safety unrelated to the implementation of the intervention plan.

Unresolved Cases: Cases may be unresolved at time of case closing for two reasons: the victim could terminate contact with the program before the intervention could be completed; and the victim could move without contacting the program or otherwise disappear without notification prior to the completion of the intervention.

Safety Outcomes Achieved: Of the sampled 56 cases, 35 or 62.5% were identified as successfully resolved because the objective of victim safety had been achieved when the case was closed. A total of 21 or 37.5 % were identified as unresolved at the time of closing because the objective of victim safety had not been achieved.

The ES Program cases included 17 with a successful outcome and 10 with an unsuccessful or unresolved outcome. Among the 10 ES Program cases that were closed prior to achieving resolution, 9 were closed at the request of the victim and one was closed because the victim could no longer be located. For the CVB Program cases, 18 reported a successful outcome at closing and 11 reported an unsuccessful outcome when the case was closed. Of the 11 CVB cases with an unsuccessful or unresolved outcome at closing, 7 cases were closed at the victims' request, and 4 were closed because the victim could no longer be located.

Of the 17 ES Program cases that were resolved at the time of case closing, 16 were resolved as a result of the program intervention and the successful resolution of one was unrelated to the program intervention. For the 18 CVB Program cases that were resolved at closing, 14 were resolved as a result of the program intervention and 4 achieved resolution unrelated to the program intervention (see Table 1).

Safety Outcomes and Legal Interventions: Of the 4 ES program cases with legal interventions, all were successfully resolved at the time of closing. It should be noted that none of these cases involved criminal acts as defined by the New York State Penal Code (see Table 2).

The legal actions in question were related to eviction proceedings in housing court. The CVB Program handled 13 cases involving criminal acts of abuse with legal interventions. Of these 10 were successfully resolved and 3 were unsuccessfully resolved at the time of case closing.

Safety Outcomes and Social Service Interventions: The ES Program provided social services to 25 cases: of these, 15 were successfully resolved at the time of closing and 10 were not successfully resolved when closed. The CVB Program provided social services to 24 cases: 15 were successfully resolved and 9 remained unresolved at the time of case closing (see Table 3).

Safety Outcomes, Types of Abuse, and Intervention Strategy

Financial Abuse: A total of 27 cases involved financial abuse. Of these 6 were served by the ES Program and 21 were served by the CVB Program. Of the 6 cases served by the ES Program, 5 (83.1%) remained unresolved at the time of the case closings, and 1 (16.7%) was resolved

TABLE 1. Safety Outcomes by Program

OUTCOME	TYPE	
	DFTA (ES)	CVB
Safety Achieved	17 (63.0%)	18 (62.1%)
Safety Not Achieved	10 (37.0%)	11 (37.9%)
Total	27 (100.0%)	29 (100.0%)

Pearson Chi Square = .005; df = 1; p = .582

TABLE 2. Legal Interventions and Safety Outcomes

Legal Intervention	TYPE	
	DFTA (ES)	CVB
Safety Achieved	4 (100.0%)	10 (76.9%)
Safety Not Achieved	0	3 (23.1%)
Total	4 (100.0%)	13 (100.0%)

Pearson Chi Square = .161; df = 1; p (1 sided) = .421

TABLE 3. Social Service Interventions and Safety Outcomes

Social Service Intervention	TYPE	
	DFTA (ES)	CVB
Safety Achieved	15 (60.0%)	15 (62.2%)
Safety Not Achieved	10 (40.0%)	9 (37.5%)
Total	25 (100.0%)	24 (100.0%)

Pearson Chi Square = 1.120; df = 1; p = .545

at closing. In comparison, of the 21 cases served by the CVB program, 14 (66.7%) were resolved at the time of case closing, and 7 (33.3%) remained unresolved. A chi-square test of association was used to identify a significant difference (p = .043) in the outcome of cases involving financial abuse, with the CVB Program, utilizing a legal strategy, significantly more successful in resolving financial abuse cases than the ES Program utilizing a social service strategy (see Table 4).

Psychological Abuse: A total of 24 cases reported psychological abuse. Of these 11 were served by the ES Program, and 13 were served by the CVB Program. Of the 11 cases served by the ES Program, 6 (54.5%)

TABLE 4. Financial Abuse, by Program, and Safety Outcome

Financial Abuse	TYPE	
	DFTA (ES)	CVB
Safety Achieved	1 (16.7%)	14 (66.6%)
Safety Not Achieved	5 (83.3%)	7 (33.3%)
Total	6 (100.0%)	21 (100.0%)

Pearson Chi Square = 1.857; df = 1; p (1 sided) = .043

TABLE 5. Psychological Abuse, by Program, and Safety Outcome

Psychological Abuse	TYPE	
	DFTA (ES)	CVB
Safety Achieved	6 (54.5%)	6 (46.2%)
Safety Not Achieved	5 (45.5%)	7 (53.8%)
Total	11 (100.0%)	13 (100.0%)

Pearson Chi Square = .155; df = 1; p (1 sided) = .5

were resolved and 5 (45.5%) were unresolved at the time of case clos-ing. Of the 13 cases served by the CVB Program, 6 (46.2%) were re-solved and 7 (53.8%) were unresolved when the cases were closed. Using a chi square test of association, no significant difference was found at the .05 level or below (see Table 5).

Physical Abuse: Of the 14 cases with reported physical abuse, 3 were served by the ES Program and all were reported as resolved at the time of case closings. Of the 11 cases served by the CVB Program, 8 (72.2%) were resolved and 3 (27.3%) were unresolved when the cases were closed. Using a chi-square test of association, no significant differences were found in case resolution for the ES and the CVB Program inter-ventions (see Table 6).

Neglect: Of the 7 cases with reported neglect in the sample, 3 were served by the ES Program: of these, 2 (66.7%) were reported as re-solved at the time of case closings and 1 (33.3%) was reported as unre-solved. Of the 4 cases served by the CVB Program, 3 (75%) were resolved and 1 (25%) remained unresolved at the time of case closings. A chi-square test of association was used to test differences using the .05 level, and no significant difference was found (see Table 7).

TABLE 6. Physical Abuse, by Program, and Safety Outcome

Physical Abuse	TYPE	
	DFTA (ES)	CVB
Safety Achieved	3 (100.0 %)	8 (72.7%)
Safety Not Achieved	0	3 (27.3%)
Total	3 (100.0%)	11 (100.0%)

Pearson Chi Square = 1.041; df = 1; p = .453

TABLE 7. Neglect, by Program and Safety Outcome

Neglect	TYPE	
	DFTA (ES)	CVB
Safety Achieved	2 (66.6 %)	3 (75%)
Safety Not Achieved	1 (33.3 %)	1 (25%)
Total	3 (100.0%)	4 (100.0%)

Pearson Chi Square = .058; df = 1; p (1 sided) = .857

Social Problems: A total of 23 cases reported social problems. Of these, 15 cases were served by the ES Program: 12 (80%) were resolved at the time of case closing, and 3 (20%) remained unresolved when the cases were closed. For those cases served by the CVB Program, social problems were not of primary concern, because all cases included criminal elements as well. Of the CVB Program cases involving social problems, 4 (50%) were resolved at the time of case closings, and 4 (50%) remained unresolved. A chi-square test of significance was used to determine that no significant difference was found between ES and CVB Program case resolution at the .05 level of significance.

Analysis of Hypotheses

Using chi-square tests of association, none of the differences were found to be statistically significant between ES and CVB Program interventions and resolved or unresolved victim safety issues at the time of case closings. This supports the null hypothesis that in cases when the abuse or neglect is defined as a crime by the New York State Penal Code, a criminal justice intervention is not more successful than a social service intervention in achieving the desired outcome of victim safety.

TABLE 8. Social Problems, by Program and Safety Outcome

Social Problems	TYPE	
	DFTA (ES)	CVB
Safety Achieved	17 (63.0%)	18 (62.1%)
Safety Not Achieved	10 (37.0%)	11 (37.9%)
Total	27 (100.0%)	29 (100.0%)

Pearson Chi Square = .005; df = 1; p = .582

It also supports the null hypothesis that when the abuse or neglect is not defined as a crime by the New York State Penal Code, a social service intervention is not more effective than a criminal justice intervention in achieving victim safety.

Research Questions: Findings

The only research question posed that elicited a finding of significant difference was: Are there differences in client safety outcomes related to type of abuse? In elder abuse cases involving financial abuse, the CVB Program was significantly more likely to achieve the objective of client safety and successfully resolve the abuse situation than was the ES Program.

SUMMARY AND IMPLICATIONS

While the Elder Service Program and the Crime Victims Board Program represent two different community-based strategies for addressing elder abuse in the community, there was no significant difference in their effectiveness based on the findings of the study conducted at Walk the Walk. While a larger number of Elder Service (ES) Program cases achieved successful resolution than those served by the Crime Victims Board (CVB) Program, the differences were not found to be statistically significant.

The more challenging nature of cases representing criminal actions on the part of an abuser may contribute to the lower number of successfully resolved CVB cases. On the other hand, both programs resolved the majority of cases reviewed in the study. It is also interesting to note that while the CVB program provided more legal interventions and engaged the criminal justice system in a manner that the ES program did not, both programs provided an almost equal number of social service interventions. This underscores the importance of social service provision in serving elder abuse victims, regardless of whether or not the identified abuse rises to the level of a crime.

The victim and abuser profile for the ES and CVB programs did not differ significantly as well. In both programs, the victims were predominantly female, the average ages of both victims and perpetrators were equivalent, and the physical functioning of victims–all of whom lived independently in the community at the time they received service from Walk the Walk–did not differ among programs.

Implications for Policy and Practice

Two significant differences between the ES and CVB Programs were identified by the study. One was that self-neglect cases were served exclusively by the ES Program. Self neglect cases are not likely to be served by crime victims programs, in the absence of an identified perpetrator. The second was that for financial abuse cases, the CVB Program was significantly more likely to achieve a successful outcome than the ES Program. This suggests that financial exploitation of older adults is most effectively addressed by crime victims programs.

Based on the findings of this study, it appears that elder abuse ranges on a continuum from self-neglect and difficulties in family relations, to abuse perpetrated by family members and others that rises to the level of a crime. Both elder service and crime victim approaches are effective in serving elder abuse victims, and the difference in service orientation between the two approaches complement one another. For example, social service approaches are clearly most valuable in addressing self-neglect cases, and crime victim approaches, based on the findings of this study, are most effective in serving financial abuse victims.

Also of significance is the finding that social service interventions are utilized regardless of whether the program focus is that of serving older victims and their families in later life, or serving elderly crime victims. This suggests the importance of social work services not only in social service programs serving elder abuse victims, but also in programs that serve older victims of crime, including family crimes. Graduate schools of social work should integrate aging and elder abuse content into the social work curriculum, and social workers who serve the elderly should seek training, including in-service training, on elder abuse and neglect. This would help to achieve both safety and justice for older victims of abuse and neglect in our communities.

Limitations and Implications for Future Research

The study included a small number of subjects, although randomly selected, and was confined to one community based agency, Walk the Walk in Queens, New York. The findings cannot be generalized beyond the programs from which study subjects were drawn. More research is needed on the comparative effectiveness of the social service and crime victim approaches to assisting elder abuse victims achieve safety in their communities.

Infusing gerontological content, including content on elder abuse and neglect, in schools of social work is critical to ensuring that older adults, including victims of elder abuse and neglect, receive needed professional social services. The John A. Hartford Foundation has recognized the need for the social work profession to prepare social work practitioners for serving older adults as our population continues to age. Professional education, informed policies, and research are all critical to achieve this goal.

REFERENCES

Bergeron, L. R. (2001). *An elder abuse case study: caregiver stress or domestic violence? You decide.* Journal of Gerontological Social Work, 34 (4), 47-63.

Brownell, P., Berman, J., & Salamone, A. (1999). *Mental health and criminal justice issues among perpetrators of elder abuse.* Journal of Elder Abuse and Neglect, 11 (4), 81-94.

Pillemer, K., & Finkelhor, D. (989). *The causes of elder abuse: caregiver stress versus problem relatives.* American Orthopsychiatric Journal, 59 (2), 179-187.

Rubin, A., & Babbie, E. (2001). *Research methods for social work, fourth edition.* Belmont, CA: Wadsworth.

Steinmetz, S. (1980). *Duty bound: elder abuse and family care.* Newbury Park, CA: Sage.

Wolf, R. S. (1999). *The criminalization of elder abuse.* Presentation: Pan American Conference '99, San Antonio, Texas, Symposium of Social Policy II, February 23, 1999.

Wolf, R. S. (2000). *A research agenda on abuse of older persons and adults with disabilities. http://www.elderabusecenter.org/research/agenda.html*

Wolf, R. S., & Pillemer, K. (2000). *Elder abuse and case outcome.* Journal of Applied Gerontology, 19 (2), 203-220.

Yin, P. (1984). *Victimization and the aged.* Springfield, Ill.: Charles C. Thomas.

Employed Women
and Their Aging Family Convoys:
A Life Course Model of Parent Care
Assessment and Intervention

M.W. Parker, LTC, DSW, BCD, LCSW
Vaughn R.A. Call, PhD
Ronald Toseland, PhD
Mark Vaitkus, LTC, PhD
Lucinda Roff, PhD
James A. Martin, PhD, BCD

M.W. Parker is affiliated with the University of Alabama, School of Social Work, Little Hall/Box 870314, University of Alabama at Birmingham, Center for Aging, Department of Geriatrics and Gerontology, Tuscaloosa, AL 35487-0314. (E-mail: Mwparker@sw.ua.edu). Vaughn R.A. Call is Chairman of the Department of Sociology at Brigham Young University, 840 SWKT, Provo, UT 84602 (E-mail: vaughn_call@byu.edu). Ronald Toseland is Professor and Director, Institute of Gerontology, School of Social Welfare, University at Albany, State University of New York, NY 12222 (E-mail: Toseland@albany.edu). Mark Vaitkus is Deputy Director, US Army Physical Fitness Research Institute, US Army War College, Carlisle, PA 17013-5050 (E-mail: Vaitkusm@awc.carlisle.army.mil). Lucinda Roff is affiliated with the University of Alabama, School of Social Work, Little Hall/Box 870314, Tuscaloosa, AL 35487-0314 (E-mail: lroff@sw.ua.edu). James A. Martin is affiliated with the Graduate School of Social Work and Social Research, Bryn Mawr, PA 19010 (E-mail: jmartin@brynmawr.edu).

Address correspondence to: Michael Parker, DSW, LTCR, BCD, LCSW, School of Social Work, University of Alabama, Center for Aging, University of Alabama at Birmingham, Little Hall, Box 870314, Tuscaloosa, AL 35487-0314 (E-mail: Mwparker@ sw.ua.edu).

[Haworth co-indexing entry note]: "Employed Women and Their Aging Family Convoys: A Life Course Model of Parent Care Assessment and Intervention." Parker, M.W. et al. Co-published simultaneously in *Journal of Gerontological Social Work* (The Haworth Social Work Practice Press, an imprint of The Haworth Press, Inc.) Vol. 40, No. 1/2, 2002, pp. 101-121; and: *Older People and Their Caregivers Across the Spectrum of Care* (ed: Judith L. Howe) The Haworth Social Work Practice Press, an imprint of The Haworth Press, Inc., 2003, pp. 101-121. Single or multiple copies of this article are available for a fee from The Haworth Document Delivery Service [1-800-HAWORTH, 9:00 a.m. - 5:00 p.m. (EST). E-mail address: docdelivery@haworthpress.com].

10.1300/J083v40n01_07

SUMMARY. Traditional models of geriatric assessment have not considered the cultural and demographic changes that have affected women's ability to provide parent care in the 21st century. The United States has the world's highest fulltime employment rate and the longest workweek. These factors have an important impact on women's ability to provide care for aging parents. A life course assessment and intervention model currently employed at the US Army and Air War Colleges that helps female and male officers prepare proactively for parent care is described. The usefulness of the model is supported by data from a longitudinal survey of the needs of military families. The life course model provides a unique framework to guide social workers who help women within and outside the armed forces to manage 21st century commitments to family and work. *[Article copies available for a fee from The Haworth Document Delivery Service: 1-800-HAWORTH. E-mail address: <docdelivery@haworthpress.com> Website: <http://www.HaworthPress.com> © 2002 by The Haworth Press, Inc. All rights reserved.]*

KEYWORDS. Parent care, life course, women and work, caregiving, midlife, caregiving assessment and intervention, caregiving resources

INTRODUCTION

More women with children work fulltime in the United States (US) (68%) than in any other nation in the world (Portugal, at 38%, has the next highest percentage of women in the work force); furthermore, fully employed Americans work more hours per year on average than workers in any other country in the world . . . almost nine full weeks more per year than the average European (Wisensale, 2001; Wisensale, 2002). As the full impact of these demographic and cultural changes is experienced, the life course theme of parent care is shared by a growing number of working women during midlife. Conflicting commitments to parent care, their nuclear and extended family, and their work and social lives make women who care for aging parents particularly vulnerable to stress and career disruption (Moen, Robison, & Fields, 2000; Coberly & Hunt, 1995; Neal, Chapman, Ingersoll-Dayton, & Emler, 1995; Creedon & Tiven, 1989).

Social scientists and historians have advocated tracking the impact of psycho-social-historical experiences and patterns on the life course transitions and trajectories of US citizens (Gade, 1991; Elder, Gimbel, &

Ivie, 1991) and developing corresponding human-resource strategies for reducing pressures on workers and their families (Parker, Fuller, Koenig, Bellis, Vaitkus, Barko, & Eitzen, 2001b; Parker, Vaitkus, Aldwin, Call, and Barko, 2000). In this paper we describe the adaptation and application of a life course model currently being used with military families. We also describe a unique program of assessment and intervention for parent care that was developed based on a longitudinal life event history survey of military officers in the US Army and Air Force. The parent care assessment and intervention program is aimed at helping women and men prepare proactively for the developmental tasks and challenges commonly associated with caring for their aging parents. We review the primary constructs of a life course framework and the advantages of this perspective for understanding caregiving by women in military and civilian settings, and we describe a parent care assessment and intervention program that is being used to assist women and men at the US Army and US Air War Colleges to plan for parent care tasks (Parker, Call, Dunkle, & Vaitkus, 2002).

Background

Contemporary families are experiencing gains in life expectancy, declining fertility rates, increased female labor-force participation, and more diverse, multigenerational family structures (Parker, Martin, & Hendrickson, 1996). At the same time, historians note that the *nuclear* family, not the three-generational family, was the 19th century norm (Hareven, 1995). They also indicate that 19th century households rarely included older family members unless they were the recipients of end of life care (Hareven, 1991). Whereas laws and public forms of assistance bind generations in today's society, social norms, and religious values bound the generations together in 19th century America (Ruggles, 1994).

Other comparisons between the 19th and 21st centuries suggest that, except for the higher incidence of divorce, contemporary families have a greater uniformity of life course sequences. Nineteenth century families experienced more frequent childhood deaths, more adult children who never married, more women who were prematurely widowed, and fewer defined periods of child-rearing, education, and leaving home (Hareven, 1995). Historians suggest that the rise of the three and four generational family structures of the late 20th and early 21st centuries in America represents a new phenomenon that lends itself to a more predictable set of life course sequences (Hareven, 1995; Call & Teachman,

1991; Marini, 1984). The historical shift to a more predictable set of life course sequences provides an opportunity for social workers and other professionals to help women and men to prepare for parent care and other age-graded developmental tasks and transitions.

It has been suggested that work and family are "greedy institutions," because both require a dedicated and time-consuming commitment from middle-aged women and men (Segal, 1986). The struggle to remain committed to both work and family is particularly difficult for women serving in the military. Competing demands have created what Moskos and Wood (1988) call a "double bind." Although there has been considerable effort during the last decade to meet the needs of military families (Martin & McClure, 2000), the fundamental conflict between vocational duty and family responsibility continues to be a pressing problem for many (Martin, Rosen, & Sparacino, 2000). Caregiving responsibilities often add considerably to the burden experienced by military and civilian women and men who have aging parents. Employers have not adequately considered the aging of the American population and its effect on career-oriented women and men who face inter-generational responsibilities (Parker et al., 2001b; Ensign, 1996; Davis & Krouze, 1994; Dellman-Jenkins, Bennett, & Brahce, 1994; Liebig, 1993; Creedon & Tiven, 1989). Many employed women at mid-life experience a "triple bind" of work, child, and parent care (Parker, Fuller, Koenig, Bellis, Vaitkus, Barko, Eitzen, & Call, 2001a; Moen, Robison, & Fields, 2000; Parker, Call, & Barko, 1999).

Social workers and other professionals have often failed to heed the social problems created by the increase in multigenerational families, elderly and disabled family members, dual career families, and single parents who work fulltime (Parker et al., 1999; Parker et al., 2001b). Social workers have responded with programs that focus on the adverse consequences of caregiving (e.g., caregiver burden, depression) (Martin, Rosen, & Sparacino, 2000; Neal et al., 1995; Krach & Brooks, 1996; Heath, 1993; Hansson & Carpenter, 1990). The positive aspects of caregiving (e.g., potential for the development of closer kinship ties, the achievement of intrinsic goals like the mastering of caregiving tasks, and the fulfillment of the commitment to "honor one's mother and father" have often been neglected because an assessment framework that would sensitize women and men to this developmental task, and encourage preparation, is lacking (Kramer & Lambert, 1999; Kramer & Kipnis, 1995; Toseland, Smith, & McCallion, 2001). Recent evidence indicates that preparing for parent care can help to prevent caregiver worry burden (Parker et al., in press; Parker et al., 2000).

An additional concern is that the impact of military service on women and their families is not well understood, despite the growing number of females who are entering fulltime military service. With a few exceptions (Parker et al., 1999; Card, 1983), life course investigations of military personnel have been limited to male, World War II veterans (e.g., Elder, 1986; Elder & Clipp, 1989; Elder, Gimbel, & Ivie, 1991; Hastings, 1991). In this article, we present life event history data from military career women at midlife, and describe a parent care intervention based on these data.

A Life Course Model

A *life course perspective* emphasizes "the ways in which people's location in the social system, the historical period in which they live, and their unique personal biography shape their experience (Parker et al., 1999)." This approach emphasizes the strong connection between individual lives and their historical context, and it provides a useful framework for addressing cultural and demographic changes that influence family and work. A life course model is the unifying framework for health promotion utilized at the US Army War College (Parker et al., 2001a; Parker et al., 2001b). In addressing the lifetime costs of military service on military families, Table 1 provides an overview of six organizing life course principles, and illustrates how each can be related to parent care among female officers. These principles have been adapted from a more comprehensive review by Parker et al. (1999).

Life course paths are mutually contingent upon the trajectories of others who are particularly significant in our lives. Overlapping life course transitions and events place military personnel and their families at increased risk for a variety of health, behavioral, and social concerns (Parker et al., 1999). For example, women on active duty may be especially vulnerable to the demands of parent care and are often forced to make transitions in their own vocational paths to accommodate changes occurring in their parents' lives (Parker, 1994).

Social support systems are composed of a network of immediate and extended family, friends, neighbors, and colleagues who provide emotional and instrumental support. For this article, we have adapted what Antonucci and Akiyama call the *convoy model of social relations*. The notion of a convoy illustrates the protective role of social support systems across the life course, and underscores the often lifelong, dynamic nature of social relationships (Antonucci & Akiyama, 1987).

TABLE 1. Life Course Principles & Parent Care Themes that Affect Military Women

Six Life Course Principles	Parent Care Themes
1. Linkages between social and psychological states form trajectories.	Most officers feel responsible for the care of their aging parents even though they may live long distances from them; therefore, late life parental care is generally considered a responsibility for adult children, and represents a socially sanctioned developmental task particularly for women.
2. Life course trajectories are embedded in social contexts.	A female officer is expected by her family to resign her commission to care for an aging parent even though her four brothers live closer.
3. Significant deviations from social pathways have negative consequences.	A female officer forced to resign her commission or who has to retire early from her military career to care for a dependent, aging family member, suffers adverse, long term vocational and financial consequences.
4. Life course trajectories are shaped by historical events.	A female officer in the US Army Reserves, the primary caregiver to her aging parents and her two children in middle school, is called to active duty during Desert Storm.
5. Life course trajectories are interdependent.	The death of one parent impacts the capacity of another parent to live independently and affects a female officer's career because she is their only child.
6. The impact of transitions is largely contingent on timing in the life course.	A female officer, who married and had children late in life, is forced to retire early from active duty because of the triple bind of work, childcare, & parent care. She and her family suffer financially later in life due to reduced retirement income.

As one experiences numerous role transitions across time, a life *trajectory* develops. People experience numerous changes in social status and personal identity as a result of this trajectory. The trajectory is a product of the interconnections of a family convoy that is aging in time, and is affected by social timetables and event-sequence histories such as education, vocation, marriage, parenthood, and parent care.

A *turning point* is a subjective change in one's life trajectory where the individual adopts a new set of roles and a fresh self-conception (Mandelbaum, 1973). Major turning points in life course trajectories frequently reflect involuntary role changes resulting from biological, psychological, social, and historical events beyond an individual's control. An account of one's life history often provides a record of changes in one's life direction (Hareven, 1991). Life history accounts also reflect one's status before or after an event. For example, the military mobilization during Operation Desert Storm resulted in family separations, occupational problems, and family financial difficulties for many reserve component service members (Martin, Rosen, & Sparacino, 2000).

Life events are identifiable life experiences or changes that require adaptation by individuals because they disrupt their coping skills (Stoller & Gibson, 2000). Life events such as marriage, the birth of a child, or taking a new job may be positive and anticipated. Others may be traumatic and unanticipated (e.g., death of a parent, spouse, or child; onset of Alzheimer's disease with a parent). Life events are not chronic in nature, though their consequences can be long-term. Most events, positive or negative, are stressful to some degree and demand the application of coping skills, although only negative life events typically have adverse effects on health. A life course perspective emphasizes the relationship between the interpretation of an event and its outcome. Thus, one might interpret a parent's stroke as the end of life or the beginning of a new life. Proactive preparation for common life events, such as the onset of parent care following a parent's stroke, increases the probability that, despite the trauma, coping with the stroke can be a positive and life enhancing experience.

To provide a practical illustration of how life course data can guide assessment and intervention, we present an application that reflects how female officers at midlife are often more vulnerable for the developmental task of parent care than male officers. We describe how life event history data were used to identify this issue, and how the life course framework facilitated the design and evaluation of an intervention to address this problem.

METHOD

The Setting

The settings for these newly developed life course programs are the US Army and US Air War Colleges, each representing the top tier of their respective military age-graded leadership school system. Selection to attend either school is an honor in that all future general officers are selected from the pool of graduates from such senior service colleges. Placements of a life course program in this kind of institution represents an important sanction of the overall purposes of life course programs. Grounding the program in a normal, age-graded vocational system, and conducting the intervention in a leadership school climate, as opposed to a psychiatric or psychological contextual setting (mental health center), has resulted in more ready acceptance of the program by senior officers.

The Army Physical Fitness Research Institute at the Army War College and the Wellness Center at the Air War College provide health screening, assessment, and intervention programs to all incoming students (Parker et al., 2001a; Parker et al., 2001b). In addition to providing health education and fitness programs to residents, the multidisciplinary team of staff and research scientists conducts applied research on the health and fitness of senior military personnel and their families who are over age 40. These centers also provide health promotional literature worldwide that targets senior military leaders (Parker et al., 2000).

Procedures

After arrival at the US Army and US Air War Colleges, officers undergo a series of multidisciplinary health screenings and assessments using state-of-the-art technology and approaches. For a three-year period (1997-1999), retrospective life history data were collected on incoming male and female officers at the US Army War College. In 2001, a longitudinal follow-up study was conducted with the 1988 and 1998 cohorts (Parker, Call, & Vaitkus, 2001). Life event history calendars were used to collect the data. A history calendar is an effective way to collect retrospective life course data, and it has the advantage of capturing both the timing and the effects of life events, transitions, turning points, and other experiences (Freedman, Thornton, Camburn, Alwin, and Young-DeMarco, 1988).

Data were collected about major life events, familial, and vocational trajectories, turning points, and experiences after graduating from high school (Parker et al., 2001b). Descriptive analyses identified the nature and timing of challenging, developmental tasks in midlife that might adversely affect officers' careers, their health, or the quality of their family lives. High probability life events and experiences were identified for each cohort group to better understand stressful situations they had faced during and after their graduation from the War College. The vast majority of officers in attendance at the US Army War College are male. Figure 1 portrays the timing and onset of major events and tasks common to male officers at midlife. Life course data describing female officers will be contrasted in the following section.

FIGURE 1. Officer Wellness Across the Life Course: Developmental Tasks in Major Life Domains

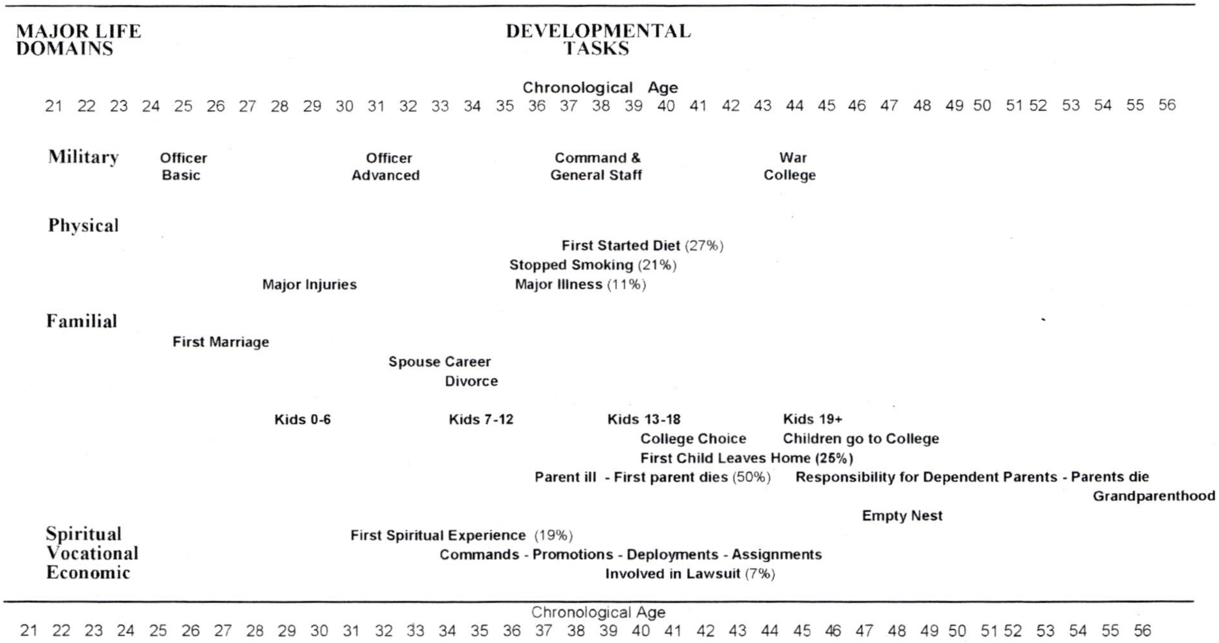

MAJOR LIFE DOMAINS

DEVELOPMENTAL TASKS

Chronological Age

21 22 23 24 25 26 27 28 29 30 31 32 33 34 35 36 37 38 39 40 41 42 43 44 45 46 47 48 49 50 51 52 53 54 55 56

Military
Officer Basic — Officer Advanced — Command & General Staff — War College

Physical
Major Injuries
Major Illness (11%)
Stopped Smoking (21%)
First Started Diet (27%)

Familial
First Marriage
Spouse Career
Divorce
Kids 0-6 — Kids 7-12 — Kids 13-18 — Kids 19+
College Choice
First Child Leaves Home (50%)
Children go to College
Parent ill - First parent dies (50%)
Responsibility for Dependent Parents - Parents die
Empty Nest
Grandparenthood

Spiritual   First Spiritual Experience (19%)
Vocational   Commands - Promotions - Deployments - Assignments
Economic   Involved in Lawsuit (7%)

Chronological Age

21 22 23 24 25 26 27 28 29 30 31 32 33 34 35 36 37 38 39 40 41 42 43 44 45 46 47 48 49 50 51 52 53 54 55 56

109

RESULTS

Life Course Justifications for Parent Care Program of Assessment and Intervention

A person's life course trajectory is interdependent on the pathways of the aging family convoy in his or her network. Although the percentages are changing, most military members are not married when they enter the military. However, the longer they remain in the military, the more likely they are to marry and have children. About sixty percent of soldiers and 80 percent of officers in the Army are married, and over 97 percent of the officers in the U. S. Army War College are married (Martin et al., 2000; Parker, Call, & Vaitkus, 2001). Based on a longitudinal survey of the '88 and '98 U.S. Army War College cohort groups, the percentage of women assigned to the Army War College doubled in the ten years from 1988 to 1998, mirroring the growing percentage of women serving on active duty (Parker, Call, & Vaitkus, 2001).

Male officers who have not experienced divorce are represented in senior leadership schools in higher numbers than those who have experienced divorce, though this pattern does not hold for female officers. Female officers are more than twice as likely to remain unmarried than their male counterparts. Though the number of married female officers attending the Army War College doubled from 1988 to 1998, married female officers are three times more likely to experience divorce than male attendees, and worry more about aging parents than do male officers (Parker, Call, & Vaitkus, 2001). Therefore, senior ranking military women may have fewer supports in their family convoys to help with parent care than males who tend to be married only once.

Women may be held to a different standard at work and at home in regard to parent care, which might account for the greater worry they report about their parents (Parker et al., 2000). As shown in Table 2, female officers, when married, do so later in life than male officers, which, in turn, delays birth of children and increases the probability of childlessness. Women having children in their late 30's or 40's are more likely to experience child and parent care simultaneously. However, married female officers have substantially fewer children than male officers, and women in this study were only slightly more likely than men to still have children living at home. Although female officers are being selected for attendance at the War College in higher numbers, and the numbers electing to marry are increasing, the higher percentage of women experiencing a divorce may reflect a gender-specific form of

TABLE 2. Life Course Events of Officers at the U.S. Army War College by Year and Sex

	Class of 1988 Active Duty			Class of 1998 Active Duty		
	Male	Female	Reserve	Male	Female	Reserve
Age at first marriage (years old)	24.5	a	24.0	24.3	27.0	24.0
First marital status						
never married	0%	50%	0%	0%	27%	3%
married to first spouse	79%	25%	70%	83%	27%	73%
divorced first spouse	20%	25%	30%	15%	46%	24%
widowed	1%	0%	0%	1%	0%	0%
Current marital status						
never married	0%	50%	0%	0%	27%	3%
married	93%	50%	100%	94%	55%	97%
divorced	6%	0%	0%	4%	18%	0%
widowed	1%	0%	0%	2%	0%	0%
Average number of children	2.3	0.0	2.4	2.2	0.4	2.0
Age at first birth (years old)	26.4	0.0	26.4	28.6	32.7	27.8
A child still at home	22%	0%	40%	86%	24%	81%
One or both parents deceased	81%	100%	80%	46%	53%	46%
Worried about parent's health (average, 1 = do not worry, 7 = worry a lot)	4.8	5.0	4.0	4.0	4.4	4.3
n^b =	135	4	10	177	17	52

[a] all data missing
[b] number of cases less for some variables

stress. While remaining married to one's first spouse is characteristic of male officers selected for the War College, women selected for attendance tend to be single, and/or divorced from the first spouse at a much higher rate. For women who are interested in having children, the biological clock of female officers serves as an additional midlife source of stress. Also, female officers are more likely to have experienced the death of one parent and the illness of a parent, which again suggest a more difficult midlife course for female career officers.

The interlocking life course pathways with parents produce additional stress for senior members of the military (Parker et al., in press). In one Army War College study, approximately one third of the officers (male and female) were not satisfied with their parents' plans for care and support during their declining years (Parker et al., 1999). About thirty percent of the officers stated that they were worried about the health of their parents, and over thirty-five percent of the officers rated their parents' health from poor to very poor. Thirty-nine percent rated the health of their in-laws as poor or worse. About two thirds of the officers have spoken to their parents about their plans associated with eldercare responsibilities, and one third were not satisfied or were very unsatisfied with their parents' plans. These officers are beginning to experience a sense of worry associated with parent care responsibilities. Male officers were almost twice as likely as female officers were to have a parent care plan. Female officers with a plan were twice as likely to report less satisfaction with the plan (Parker, Call, & Vaitkus, 2001).

In addition to multiple career pathways, military officers face elder care issues that overlap with important transitions into senior command positions (Parker et al., 2000). About half the male and female officers at the Army War College still have both parents living and more than 80 percent have at least one parent still living (Parker et al., 1999). More than half of the married officers still have both in-laws, and over 80 percent of them have at least one living in-law.

Military families represent one of the largest groups of people who live long distances from their parents and, therefore, have fewer opportunities to visit parents and extended family members. On average, members of the 1998 cohort lived 1,000 miles or more from their aging parents and in-laws. Military families find distance complicates eldercare responsibilities because of the special demands and traditions of military life (Parker et al., in press; Parker, Call, & Vaitkus, 2001; Parker & Call, 2000). In general, military families do not have the same control or influence over the location and nature of their work as do most civilians, and military housing is seldom adequate to permit frail parents to co-reside with them (Parker et al., 2000. Furthermore, the health status of parents and their geographic location are not factors considered in the assignment of military personnel (Parker et al., 2001). Only when elderly parents of active duty personnel are legally considered "dependents" are they given consideration in relocations, medical care, and other policy-related matters (Parker et al., 1999). Military operational deployments may last for many months and effectively remove the service member from any participation in parent care. Thus, the mobility, distance from parents, and residential limitations greatly restrict parent care arrangements that military personnel can make, and make coping with parent care situations potentially more stressful. This is particularly true for senior officers who assume a major command of an organization or unit.

Although the focus of this study is on active duty female officers, wives of male officers frequently serve in caregiving roles with their husbands' parents. Because women are usually the primary caregivers, they are likely to experience more stress than their husbands, particularly during overseas assignments and when limited housing arrangements reduce options. As a result, many male officers resort to contributing cash toward their parents' care because other options are not available or viable (Parker et al., in press).

The US Army War College research underscores the importance of examining the invisible "stress and anguish" of female (and male) officers who are precluded from visiting their parents by distance or assignment situations (Parker et al., in press). This research suggests that officers who are long distance caregivers typically cope with worry by contacting their parents more often by phone, mail, or email. The research also indicates that officers who are satisfied with parent-care plans experience significantly less stress associated with caregiving. Female officers, male officers prone to anger, and officers who have a history of assisting their parents with health care problems are more likely to experience stress and worry about parent care than other officers, and, therefore, are in greater need of assistance. Similarly, Parker et al. (in press) explored variables that influence worry and parent contact among military families at the US Army War College using data collected from 268 U.S. Army officers aged 40-49. A structural equation model showed that gender, previous parental illness, prior parent care experience, parent's age, number of siblings, and the tendency to have an angry temperament all contribute to officer worry. Officer satisfaction with a parent care plan was inversely related to officer worry. The finding that satisfaction with parents' later life plans reduces children's worry over their parent's well being, underscores the importance of adult children discussing their parents' late life plans.

Parker et al. (2000) have suggested that military officers need a written plan that addresses current and future parent care needs. It should identify gaps in medical insurance, help promote successful aging practices, identify family, Internet, and community resources for care, sibling caregiving responsibilities, and parent preferences for the type of care they would like to receive. The plan should also include legal and financial documents (e.g., will, location of important legal documents, durable power of attorney, and living will).

The Parent Care Readiness Assessment

In order to respond to the lack of preparation for parent care revealed from the life event history analysis, a Parent Care Readiness Assessment and intervention were developed for trial testing as a part of an overall Wellness Program at the US Air War College. Senior leadership schools were targeted as sites to prepare students for the developmental task of 'honoring one's aging mother and father' because parent care issues are more likely to affect those who are 35 years old or older (Parker et al., 2001b). The goals of the intervention are to develop a program that helps officers prepare for parent care, and minimize their risks (e.g., reduced performance and role conflict). The specific purpose of the long-distance parent care project is to conduct and evaluate a psycho-social educational intervention aimed at helping at risk military careerists who tend to live long distances from their parents complete specific tasks to prepare them for the provision of care for their parent(s). The intervention includes a two-hour workshop, access to a military web site developed specifically for the purpose of assisting military family, expert advice, and state of the art resource materials related to long-term care decision making.

The Parent Care Readiness Assessment contains over 50 specific tasks associated with parent care. Many of these are listed in Table 3. Tasks are organized into categories in keeping with the four primary themes of the intervention: (1) medical, (2) legal/financial, (3) social/familial, and (4) spiritual/emotional. Officers are asked: to assess the level of importance of each task; to indicate whether they have completed the task; to report how satisfied they are with the completed task; and, if they have not completed the task, to indicate when they plan to complete the task. Tasks range from "completion of a durable power of attorney" (legal-financial category) to "organizing a family meeting" to "discussing parent care responsibilities and roles" (social-familial category).

IMPLICATIONS

Maintaining contact and providing care to aging parents represents a midlife developmental task for civilians and career military personnel alike. Unfortunately, the military has lagged behind in understanding the psychological and vocational effects of parent care, and in designing programs to assist career military personnel with the challenges of this

TABLE 3. Parent Care Categories and Sample Associated Tasks

Legal-Financial Tasks	Medical Tasks	Social-Familial Tasks	Spiritual-Emotional Tasks
Discuss with your parents the advantages of completing and the consequences of neglecting to complete each of the following documents related to estate dispersion and management, advance directives, etc.	Discuss with your parents how involved or knowledgeable he or she would like for you to be about health condition, diagnoses, medications, and functional status.	Together with your spouse clarify your own values about where parents' care fits with your other life responsibilities.	Make peace with your parents.
Estate dispersion: • Will • Joint Ownership & Tenancy • Trust/Revocable living trust • Durable Power of Attorney • Preferred possession list	Obtain access to results of comprehensive geriatric assessment.	Assess your relationship with your parents, siblings and other relatives who would realistically be an acceptable resource for your parent's care.	Secure a video or oral history from your parents.
Advance Directives • Health care proxy • Do not resuscitate orders • Living Will	Log information acquired from medical appointments	Convene a family conference to formulate plans. Address who can and will do what, when, and how for your parents.	Investigate the nature of religious programs for seniors available for your parents in their home community
Secure accessible location of legal documents.	Compile a list of parents' health care providers & telephone #s.	Make sure that you know the name, address, email, and phone number of at least three people who live near your parents and who you could telephone if you could not reach your parents.	Establish an active prayer life with your parents, and cultivate prayer time with them by phone.
Rule out legal dependency of parents as a way to secure medical and treatment options.	Compile a list of current medications and obtain a copy of current medical records.	Develop a plan that would allow your parent to remain safely in their home and a plan that includes a move to another location if this becomes necessary.	Identify your parents' wishes for funeral and burial or cremation. If pre-need plans have been made, locate the documentation.

TABLE 3 (continued)

Legal-Financial Tasks	Medical Tasks	Social-Familial Tasks	Spiritual-Emotional Tasks
Assist parents in identifying assets, liabilities, income, and expenses.	Verify that primary care doctor or pharmacist is monitoring medications.	Discuss with your parent the possibility of a "panic button" service.	Establish a reliable point of contact of at least one member of your parents' church, synagogue, mosque, or religious organization.
Check parent's social security care for accuracy & review parents' credit history. If applicable, make sure mother has access to joint or separate credit.	Maintain a list of local emergency service providers (addresses, telephone #s).	Understand the long-term care options available in your parent's home community (living options, in and out of home services).	Encourage your parents to complete a codicil to the will that represents what s(he) would like to say to the next generation.
Investigate the costs of long term care scenarios (e.g., long term care insurance, savings).	Compile a list of services and programs that encourage successful aging practices and suggest appropriate parental involvement.	Evaluate the safety of your parent's home situation (falls, isolation, scams), and employ appropriate strategies to increase safety.	Understand hospice and palliative care so as to assist your parents in the death and dying process if it becomes necessary.
Determine the full extent of your parent's health/life insurance coverage, as well as Medicare and Medicaid entitlements.	Identify signs that indicate your parent can not live independently.	Discuss the feasibility of a driving assessment.	Encourage your parents' faith.

task (e.g., Ensign, 1996; Coberly & Hunt, 1995; Davis & Krouze, 1994; Dellman-Jenkins, Bennett, & Brahce, 1994; Creedon & Tiven, 1989). This is particularly problematic for senior career women in the military who tend to be single, or divorced at higher percentages than male counterparts. Because women are more likely to be primary caregivers, female officers may be more vulnerable than male officers to the midlife stressors associated with the vocational and psychological effects of parent care.

Though civilian organizations have responded with a variety of programs to assist civilian employees and to minimize the adverse psychological and vocational consequences that often accompany filial responsibilities (Ensign, 1996; Walter, 1996; Krach & Brooks, 1996; Coberly & Hunt, 1995; Davis & Krouze, 1994; Creedon & Tiven, 1993; Dellman-Jenkins et al., 1994; Liebig, 1993; Wilson, Nippes, Simson, & Mahovich, 1993; Toseland & Smith, 2001; Toseland, Smith, and McCallion, 2001; Winfield, 1987), the effects of parent care on the welfare of military personnel have not been systematically studied, nor have remedies been recommended or assessed as they have been with civilian workers (Parker et al., 2000).

A major limitation of this study is the small sample size of female officers. Plans are underway to conduct similar studies with a larger sample of women (enlisted and officer) at midlife in the military. Until these studies are completed, these results should be considered preliminary. Nevertheless, the results underscore the value of a life course perspective in identifying challenges associated with particular life stages, especially when these issues are related to demographic and cultural changes. In this paper, data from two cohorts of officers were used as the basis for the design of a parent care assessment and intervention program in a military setting.

The timing of social and family events should be taken into account in the design of health promotion and family related programs because some life events are predictable and sensitive to gender issues (e.g., young adult > marriage; midlife > parent care, remarriage). In response to these predictable events that often reflect a developmental task, organizational programs and policies can be designed from a life course, age-graded perspective to assist and prepare individuals and families for these high probability life events and attendant challenges. In the future, intervention programs based on life event history analysis may reveal systemically when people are at risk for divorce, financial problems, parenting challenges, or filial responsibilities. The impact of these factors on vocational retention, performance, and personal and family health, can be assessed for women and men. If the parent care intervention program based on life course data currently in a clinical trial development phase at the US Air War College proves effective, then broader applications of this intervention should be considered in preparing women (and men) for the task of parent care in other military and civilian settings.

REFERENCES

Abel, E. (1991). *Who cares for the elderly? Public policy and the experience of adult daughters.* Philadelphia: Temple University Press.

Anthony, J. (1995). Your aging parents: Documenting their wishes. *American Health,* 109: 58-61.

Antonucci, T., & Akiyama, H. (1987). Social networks in adult life and a preliminary examination of the convoy model. *Journal of Gerontology.* 42: 519-27.

Bell, B.D. (1991). The impact of Operation Desert Shield/Storm on Army Families: A summary of findings to date. 53rd Annual Conference of the National Council on Family Relations.

Call, V.R., Teachman, J.D. (1991). Military service and disruption of the family life course. *Military Psychology* 3: 233-251.

Call, V.R.A., & J.D. Teachman. (1991). Military service and stability in the family life course. *Military Psychology* 3(4), 233-250.

Card, J.J. (1983). *Lives after Vietnam: The personal impact of military service.* Lexington, MA Lexington Books.

Cashin, Joan E. (2000). Households, Kinfolk and absent Teenagers: The Demographic Transition in the Old South. *Journal of Family History* 25(2): 55-71.

Coberly, S., & Hunt, G. G. (1995). *The Metlife Study of employer costs for Working Caregivers.* Washington, DC: Washington Business Group on Health.

Coolbaugh, K., & Rosenthal A. (1992). *Family Separations in the Army.* (Technical Report 964) Alexandria, VA: US Army Research Institute for the Behavioral and Social Sciences (AD A258-274).

Creedon, M. Al, & Tiven, M. (1989). *Elder Care in the Workplace.* National Council on the Aging & National Association of State Units on Aging, Washington, DC.

Davis, E., & Krouze, M. K. (1994). Maturing benefit: Eldercare after a decade, *Employee Benefits Journal,* 19(3): 16-20.

Dellman-Jenkins, M., Bennett, J. M., & Brahce, C. I. (1994). Shaping the corporate response to workers with eldercare commitments: Considerations for gerontologists. *Educational Gerontology,* 20(4): 395-405.

Elder, G.H. (1986). Military times and turning points in men's lives. *Developmental Psychology,* no. 22: 233-245.

Elder, G. H. (1987). War mobilization and life course: A cohort of World War II. *Sociological Forum,* no. 2: 449-472.

Elder, G.H. Jr. & Clipp, E.C. (1989). Combat experience and emotional health: Impairment and resilience in later life. *Journal of Personality,* no. 57: 311-341.

Elder, G. H. (1988a). Combat experience, comradeship, and psychological health. In *Human adaptation to extreme stress: From the Holocaust to Vietnam*, edited by J.P. Harel, Z. Wilson, B. Kahana, 226-273. New York: Plenum.

Elder, G. H. (1988b). Wartime losses and social bonding: Influences across 40 years in men's lives. *Psychiatry*, no. 51: 177-197.

Elder, G.H. Jr., Gimbel, C., Ivie, R. (1991). Turning points in life: The case of military service and war. *Military Psychology*, no. 3: 215-231.

Elder, G.H. Jr., Pavalko, E.K.; Hastings, T.J. (1991). Talent, history and the fulfillment of promise. *Psychiatry* 54: 251-267.

Elder, G.H., Bailey, S.L. (1988). The timing of military service in men's lives. In *Social Stress and Family Development*, edited by D.M. Aldous & J. Klein, 157-174. New York: Guilford Press.

Ensign, D. A. (1996). Integrated employee assistance program response to aging issues. *Ageing International*. 23 (fall): 38-52.

Etheridge, R. (1989). *Family Factors Affecting Retention: A Review of the Literature*. Alexandria, VA: U.S. Army Research Institute for the Behavioral and Social Sciences.

Fligstein, N. (1976). *The GI Bill: Its effects on the educational and occupational attainments of U.S. males, 1940-1973*. Madison, WI: University of Wisconsin Center for Demography and Ecology.

Freeman, D., Thornton, A., Camburn, D., Alwin, D., & Young-DeMarco, L. (1988). The Life history calendar: A technique for collecting retrospective data. *Sociological Methodology*. New York.

Gade, P. (1991). Military service and the life-course perspective: A turning point for military personnel research. *Military Psychology* 3: 187-200.

Hansson, R. O., & Carpenter, B. N. (1990). Relational competence and adjustment in older adults: Implications for the demands of aging. In M.A.P. Stephens, J.H. Crowther, S.E. Hobfoll, & D. Tennenbaum (Eds.) *Stress and coping in later-life families*. 131-151. New York: Hemisphere Publishing.

Hareven, T.K. (1995). *Family time and industrial time*. New York: Cambridge University Press.

Hareven, T. K. (1991). The history of the family and the complexity of social change. *American Historical Review*. 96: 95-124.

Hastings, T.J. (1991). The Stanford-Terman study revisited: Postwar emotional health of World War II Veterans. *Military Psychology*, no. 3: 201-214.

Havighurst, R.J., Baughman, J.W., Burgess, E.W., Eaton, W.H. (1951). *The American veteran back home*. New York: Longsman, Green.

Heath, A. (1993). *Long distance caregiving: A survival guide for far away caregivers*, New York: American Source Books.

Krach, P., & Heath, J. A. (1996). Identifying the responsibilities and needs of working adults who are primary caregivers. *Journal of Gerontological Nursing*, 21(10): 41-50.

Kramer, B. J. (1997). Differential predictors of strain and gain among husbands caring for wives with dementia. *The Gerontologist*, 37, 239-249.

Kramer, B. J., & Lambert, J. D. (1999). Caregiving as a lifecourse transition among older husbands: A prospective study. *The Gerontologist*. 39: 658-667.

Kramer, B. J., & Kipnis, S. (1995). Eldercare and work role conflict: Toward an understanding of gender differences in caregiver burden. *The Gerontologist.* 35: 340-348.

Liebig, P. S. (1993). Factors affecting the development of employer-sponsored eldercare programs: Implications for employed caregivers. *Journal of women and aging.* 5(1): 59-78.

Lund, D.A., Caserta, M.S., Dimond, M. (1993). The course of spousal bereavement in later life. In *Handbook of Bereavement*, Stroebe, W., and Hanson, R., 240-254. Cambridge: Cambridge University Press.

Magnum, S.; Ball, D. (1987). Military skill training: Some evidence for transferability. *Armed Forces and Society* 5: 219-242.

Mandelbaum, D. G. (1973). The study of life history: Gandhi. *Current Anthropology*, no. 14: 177-196.

Marini, M. (1984) The order of events in the transition to adulthood. *Sociology of Education* 57, 63-84.

Martin, J.A., Rosen, L.N., & Sparacino, L.R. (2000). *The military family: A practice guide for human service providers.* Westport, Connecticut: Praeger.

Martin, James A. (2000). Afterword. In *The Military Family: A Practice Guide for Human Service Providers*, edited by James A.; Rosen Martin, Lenora N.; Sparacino, Linette R., 257-269. Westport, Ct.: Praeger.

Martin, James A.; McClure, Peggy. (2000). Today's Active Duty Military Family: The Evolving Challenges of Military Family Life. In *The Military Family: A Practice Guide for Human Service Providers*, edited by James A. Martin; Rosen, Lenora N.; Sparacino, Linette R., 3-23. Westport, CT.: Praeger.

Martin, James A.; Rosen, Leora N.; Sparacino, Linette R., Ed. *The Military Family: A Practice Guide for Human Service Providers.* Westport, CT: Praeger, 2000.

Moen, P., Robison, J., & Fields, V. (2000). Women's work and caregiving roles: A life course approach. In *Worlds of Difference: Inequality in the Aging Experience*, 3rd Ed., Eds. Stoller, E. P. and Gibson, R. C. Thousand Oaks, CA: Pine Forge Press.

Moskos, C.C.; Wood, F.R. (1988). *The Military: More than just a job?* Washington, DC: Pergamon-Brassy's.

Neal, M., Chapman, M., Ingersoll-Dayton, B., & Emler, A. (1995). *Balancing Work and Care Giving for Children, Adults, and Elders.* London: Sage Publication.

Parker, M. W., Call, V. R., Dunkel, R., & Vaitkus, M. (In press). " 'Out of sight' but not 'Out of Mind': Parent contact and worry among senior ranking male officers in the military who live long distances from parents." *Military Psychology.*

Parker, M. W., Fuller, G. F., Koenig, H. G., Vaitkus, M. A., Bellis, J. M., Barko, W. F., Eitzen, J., & Call, V. R. (2001a). Soldier and family wellness across the life course: A developmental model of successful aging, spirituality, and health promotion, Part I. *Military Medicine*, 166 (6): 485-489.

Parker, M., Fuller, G., Koenig, H., Bellis, J., Vaitkus, M., Barko, W., and Eitzen, J. (2001b). Soldier and Family Wellness across the Life course: A Developmental Model of Successful Aging, Spirituality and Health Promotion, Part II, *Military Medicine*, 166 (7), 561-570.

Parker, M., Call, V., & Vaitkus, M. (2001). *White Paper II: Contemporary Military Leaders and their Aging Family Convoy: A Life Course Study of health, family, vocation & Spirituality.* Carlisle, PA. US Army War College.

Parker, M. W., Vaitkus, M. A., Aldwin, C., Call, V., & Barko, W. (2000). Senior leader preparation for mid-life challenges. In W. Barko & M. Vaitkus (Eds.), *The Army War College guide to executive health and fitness (pp. 23-40).* Carlisle, PA: AWC Press.

Parker, M.W., Call, V. R., & Barko, W. F. (1999). Officer wellness across the life course. In J. G. Daley (Ed.), *Military social work (pp. 255-274). New York:* The Haworth Press, New York.

Parker, M.W., & Call, V. (1999). Soldiers and Families across the life course, Presentation at Gerontological Society's Annual Meeting, November 21, San Francisco, CA.

Parker, M. W., Martin, S., & Hendrickson, K. (1996). Eldercare, an issue that's 'come of age' for military families, *Military Family Research Digest*, 2(3), 9-11.

Parker, M.W. (1994). Eldercare, An issue that's 'come of age' for military families. Paper presented at *US Army, Europe and Seventh Army Medical Department Annual Conference*, Garmisch, Germany, April.

Parker, M.W., Achenbaum, W.A., Fuller, G.F., & Fay, W.P. (1994-1995). Aging Successfully: The example of Robert E. Lee. *Parameters* : 2: 99-113.

Pavalko, E.K., & Elder, G.H. Jr. (1990). World War II and divorce: A life-course perspective. *American Journal of Sociology*, no. 5: 1213-1234.

Rowe, J.W., & Kahn, R.L. (1998). *Successful Aging*. New York: Pantheon/Random House.

Ruggles, Steven. (1994). The Transformation of American Family Structure. *American Historical Review* 99: 103-128.

Segal, M.W. (1986). The Military and the family as greedy institutions. *Armed Forces and Society* 113: 9-38.

Segal, M.W., & Harris, J.J. (1993). What We Know About Army Families (Special Report 21)." Alexandria VA: U.S. Army Research Institute for the Behavioral and Social Sciences.

Stoller, E.P.; Gibson, R.C. (2000). *World of Difference: Inequality in the Aging Experience*. 3rd Ed. London: Pine Forge Press.

Teachman, J.D., & Call, V.R. (1996). The Effect of Military Service on Educational, Occupational and Income Attainments. *Social Science Research* 25: 1-31.

Toseland, R., Smith, G., & McCallion, P. (2001). Helping Family Caregivers. In Gitterman (Ed.), *Handbook of social work practice with vulnerable and Resilient populations* (2nd Ed.) 548-581. NY: Columbia University Press.

Toseland, R., & Smith, T. (2001). *Supporting Caregivers Through Education and Training*. A technical assistance monograph prepared for the National Family Caregiver Support Program Initiative of the U.S. Administration on Aging.

Walter, K. (1996). Elder care obligations challenge the next generation. *HR Magazine*, 41(7), 98-100.

Williams, R., & Williams, V. (1994). *Anger kills*. New York: HarperCollins.

Wilson, L. B., Nippes, J. K., Simson, S., & Mahovich, P. (1993). Status of employee caregiver benefits. *Employee Benefits Journal*, 18(1), 10-12.

Winfield, F. E. (1987). Workplace solutions for women under eldercare pressure. *Personnel*, 64(7), 31-39.

Wisensale. S. (2001). *Family leave policy: The political economy of work and family in America*. Armonk, NY: M.E. Sharpe.

Wisensale, S. (2002). The inescapable balancing act: Work, family, and caregiving. *The Gerontologist*. 42 (3): 421-424.

FROM THE WORLD OF PRACTICE

The Friendly Companion Program

Lisa Marmor Goldman, ACSW

SUMMARY. The Friendly Companion Program was initiated in May of 1999 to enhance social support for VAMC Northport Nursing Home residents who have infrequent or no visitation by family, friends, or significant others. Friendly Companions are adult and youth volunteers who make a commitment to visit residents on a regular basis. The resulting relationship appears to stimulate increased social interaction and maximize quality of life for nursing home residents. The program is considered part of the overall patient clinical care with multi-disciplinary involvement for volunteer training, patient referral, and evaluation by staff and patients. Social Work Performance Improvement measures and outcomes are discussed. *[Article copies available for a fee from The Haworth Document Delivery Service: 1-800-HAWORTH. E-mail address: <docdelivery@haworthpress.com> Website: <http://www.HaworthPress.com> © 2002 by The Haworth Press, Inc. All rights reserved.]*

[Haworth co-indexing entry note]: "The Friendly Companion Program." Goldman, Lisa Marmor. Co-published simultaneously in *Journal of Gerontological Social Work* (The Haworth Social Work Practice Press, an imprint of The Haworth Press, Inc.) Vol. 40, No. 1/2, 2002, pp. 123-133; and: *Older People and Their Caregivers Across the Spectrum of Care* (ed: Judith L. Howe) The Haworth Social Work Practice Press, an imprint of The Haworth Press, Inc., 2003, pp. 123-133. Single or multiple copies of this article are available for a fee from The Haworth Document Delivery Service [1-800-HAWORTH, 9:00 a.m. - 5:00 p.m. (EST). E-mail address: docdelivery@haworthpress.com].

10.1300/J083v40n01_08

KEYWORDS. Nursing home, visitors, social interaction, volunteers, quality of life, Friendly Companion, Performance Improvement, social isolation, institutionalized elders, cohesive climate

Creating an environment for nursing home residents which stimulates maximum social support and opportunity for interaction with others appears to be an important factor to adjustment and overall satisfaction. It is well documented in the literature that social networks and support are important to the health and well being of older people (Patterson, 1995). A significant source of support that links the nursing home resident to family and community is the presence of visitors. Research findings have indicated that the presence of visitors appears to have a therapeutic influence on patient well being (Greene, 1982) and appears to result in a more positive nursing home experience (Gueldner et al., 2001). It is also noted, however, that lack of visitors and isolation from the outside community remains a reality for a large number of nursing home residents (Gueldner et al., 2001). Port et al. (2001) note in their findings that nursing home patients with dementia receive less visitors, and all contact from family and friends decreased by approximately half following nursing home admission. Lack of intimate relationships with significant others in the nursing home environment is noted by Hicks (2000) to be a significant factor contributing to loneliness, along with increased dependency and loss. As noted in a review of literature by Windriver (1993), research findings indicate that social isolation and resulting loneliness may result in feelings of hopelessness, inability to perform independent living, and physical deterioration for institutionalized elders. Therefore, it remains essential to creatively look at multi-disciplinary programming within the nursing home setting to build supports and meaningful social interaction into daily lives of residents.

The Northport VA Friendly Companion Program was established by Social Work Service in May of 1999 to maximize the quality of life and social enrichment for veteran residents in the Nursing Home Care Units who have infrequent or no visitation by family, friends, or significant others. Friendly Companion volunteers are comprised of adults and high school age youth that make a commitment to visit residents on a regular basis to provide companionship and friendly visits, thereby enhancing opportunities for interpersonal interaction, stimulation, and contact with others. While decreasing loneliness, boredom, and feelings of isolation, companionship provided by volunteers can further validate and affirm self worth through continued presence, interest in the resident, and the positive relationship that is formed. In a study evaluating adjustment to life in a nursing home, Patterson (1995) noted that residents mentioned informal talking and visits as helpful. While offered primarily by family and other residents, residents did not care who was the source. For residents new to the nursing home environment, Friendly Companion volunteers can provide an additional source of support, and assist with transition to the unit by providing increased socialization through individual and group activities, and helping to facilitate communication and interaction with other residents. Volunteers also aid in the delivery of services provided by Nursing Home Care Unit staff by doing concrete tasks, such as letter writing or running errands, which may free staff to focus on patient care functions.

PROGRAM DESCRIPTION

The Social Work Coordinator met initially with the Voluntary Service Chief and staff to present the idea, gain support, and organize a system for volunteer referrals. The support of Voluntary Service has been essential to the success of this program by providing an ongoing base of referrals. The idea was also initially presented to Nursing Management staff, and presented at clinical staff meetings as the Friendly Companion Program is considered part of the overall clinical care with multi-disciplinary involvement for volunteer training, patient referral, and evaluation.

The nursing home Interdisciplinary Team assesses patients for participation in the Friendly Companion Program based on criteria of minimal visits by family or significant others, ability to respond, willingness to participate, and need for enhanced social interaction. Participation in the program is noted on the individual patient careplan, and documented in the patient's medical record. Once the team generates a referral, the Social Work Coordinator meets with the patient to determine interest, and to conduct further assessment of quality of life domains and area for improved satisfaction. Often, residents identify such areas as feelings of loneliness, loss of independence, loss of family contacts, wanting to be useful and appreciated by others. Preferences regarding gender/age of volunteer and how time will be spent are explored to assist the social work coordinator in determining assignment of volunteer based on attributes, interest and skill. The Interdisciplinary Team reviews patient involvement in the program on a quarterly basis, noting any improvements toward patient goals as a result of participation in the program.

A formal procedure for screening potential volunteers referred by Voluntary Service was developed by the Social Work Coordinator that includes a thorough initial interview which evaluates prospective volunteers along criteria such as interest, past experience, qualities such as flexibility, ability to listen, interact, be supportive, and willingness to accept training. The objective for this screening is to determine suitability and potential for satisfaction with this assignment. Volunteer retention remains an important area of consideration, as residents who participate in the program form a relationship that becomes an important part of their life and something to look forward to. The goal is to provide an experience that is mutually satisfying to both volunteer and resident. It appears that the match of resident and volunteer is critical to the success of the relationship, and in addition to assessing for patient needs, volunteer needs must be carefully assessed. Potential volunteers are evaluated for preferences regarding level of patient functioning, and particular skills and interest. As noted in the Friendly Companion Program Flowchart, the volunteer is referred back to Voluntary Service if the individual is not well suited for this type of assignment (see Figure 1).

Once accepted as a Friendly Companion Volunteer, the individual is required to participate in a multi-disciplinary orientation and training which is organized by the Social Work Coordinator. Nursing Home staff are involved in the training and meet with volunteers to discuss topics specific to their service. These topics include: Active Listening and Effective Communication, which is presented by Psychology Service staff; Ideas for How to Spend Time, with input from Recreation Therapy Staff; Nursing Home Do's and Don'ts, What to Expect, with assistance from Nursing staff; and Patient Confidentiality as presented by the Social Work Coordinator. The Social Work Coordinator works with Voluntary Service to orient volunteers to particulars such as obtaining a badge, logging in hours, and maintaining a book to record Friendly Companion visits. A log has been developed to maintain individual records of how time is spent for each patient. The Social Work Coordinator discusses individual assignments with volunteers, and provides intensive supervision once the volunteer begins, and is provided as needed once the volunteer is comfortable, which typically takes a few weeks. The Social Work Coordinator continues to provide education regarding patient needs and abilities, and provides direction as needed to volunteers. It is important to note that not all assignments work well, and volunteers are asked for feedback regarding comfort

FIGURE 1. Friendly Companion Program Flow Chart

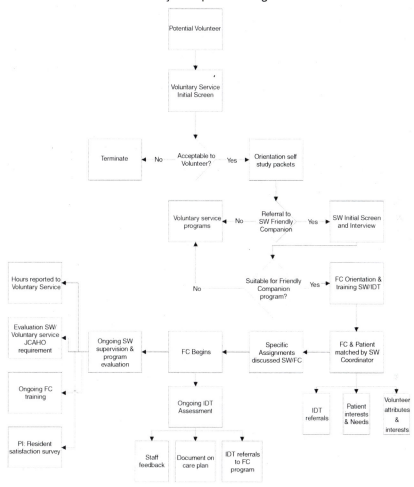

level with individual patients. In some cases, it works better to reassign volunteers to a different patient. Volunteers need to feel useful and appreciated, and the success of the relationship is critical to whether this will result in a satisfying experience.

Volunteers are typically assigned between 2-5 patients to visit individually per week, depending on time and interest. Most volunteers visit on a once per week basis, though some choose to visit more frequently. For volunteers who express willingness to meet with more cognitively impaired patients, assignments will also include higher functioning patients to ensure that some relationships can be formed which will be satisfying and mutual. Some volunteers have additionally chosen to have groups with residents to further stimulate social interaction among peers. Programs are individualized based on patient needs and interests of the volunteers. Volunteers who participate in this program range from retired individuals who wish to "give something back" to high school age youth who initially seek volunteer work to satisfy school requirements for community service. Many of these youths have continued beyond the requirement, with some coming back during college breaks to visit. In addition to continued recruitment efforts by Voluntary Service, a significant source of referrals for potential volunteers have also been generated from Chaplain Service. The Social Work Coordinator has also made presentations at Veterans Administration Voluntary Service meetings in an effort to publicize the program. All potential volunteers are directed to Voluntary Service for initial screening. Please refer to the Friendly Companion Flowchart to note organization of the Friendly Companion Program.

PROGRAM EVALUATION

To date, approximately 49% of Nursing Home residents have participated in the Friendly Companion Program, which represents all those found eligible to participate, based on criteria of limited visits from family and others, willingness to participate, and ability to respond with at least eye contact. Residents who participate in the Friendly Companion program are asked to participate in a Friendly Companion Resident Satisfaction Survey developed to provide feedback for program improvement. Questions included in the survey explore satisfaction with the program, preferences regarding age and gender of volunteer, activities, and suggestions for improvements. The Social Work Coordinator presents ongoing Performance Improvement indicators to the Social Work Performance Improvement Committee, and Extended Care Performance Improvement Committee every six months. To date, 100% of veterans who were able to complete the survey responded "yes" to the question "Do you enjoy the visits by Friendly Companion Volunteers?" All residents who have participated in the program report that they look forward to weekly visits with Friendly Companion Volunteers, and staff have noted a decrease in symptoms of anxiety and depression for some residents as a result of increased socialization and participation in the program. Resident comments have included "it takes my mind off myself," "with people to talk to, I feel better," and "it shows you we are not forgotten and still a part of everything."

As per results of Social Work Performance Improvement Indicators, about 95% of residents whom participate in the program have identified conversation as the preferred use of time, with playing board games as second choice. Several residents also identified reading the paper, writing letters, and sharing music as other favorite activities to do with Friendly Companion volunteers. Residents who participate in this program appear to demonstrate an increase in overall social interaction with peers and interest in participation in other unit activities. In a study by Mitchell and Kemp (2000), it is noted that cohesion, defined as an index of social climate, was the strongest predictor of overall quality of life for older adults in assisted living facilities. It seems that the presence of volunteers, coordination of staff to support the volunteers, and increased interaction among peers offers a positive cohesive climate for Nursing Home residents. It also appears in some cases, the Friendly Companion takes on the role of surrogate family, as they express emotional connection and concern for the well being of the patient. It is important to note that Social Work does provide additional support to volunteers in cases where the patient passes. All are invited to attend a Memorial Service held in the Nursing Home for staff, family, and interested others. During a Memorial Service held in the Nursing Home for a veteran that passed, his Friendly Companion offered a Spontaneous speech, referring to the veteran as being like an 'uncle' to him. Friendly Companions also provide an additional source of information and feedback about the patient, which is useful for the treatment team in evaluating patient care and treatment needs. Inter-disciplinary staff has verbalized support for this program, noting the positive influence for patients and the creative work by volunteers. All Nursing Home staff feel strongly that this program provides an essential service and has improved quality of life for Nursing Home patients.

Several volunteers have made notable and creative contributions. One Friendly Companion organized a trip to the beach for a resident who was a former lifeguard with the approval of medical staff, and also invited the resident home for Thanksgiving dinner. Immediately prior to his death, this veteran still reminisced with staff about his last visit to the beach. Other volunteers have sent crates of fruit from Florida, postcards and letters while on vacation, which pleases residents who feel someone is thinking of them. One Friendly Companion creatively matches less verbal patients with one another in checker games to increase social interaction, while another provides a weekly coffee group to promote social interaction. Recently, it was noted by Psychology staff that one of the more nonverbal and less responsive residents was engaged in discussion of poetry with his Friendly Companion during a visit, which appeared to stimulate memories and a former interest of the veteran. Patients appear to become emotionally attached to the Friendly Companions, and they often wait for visits. For one 79-year-old male diagnosed with schizophrenia, the Friendly Companion visit has become the focus of his week. Prior to his involvement in the program, he remained in his room isolated for much of the day, by choice. Since his involvement for the past two years, he has become interested in going outside to get "fresh air" where he anticipates his visits. He eagerly talks about his Companion and the visits to staff, and it seems to give him something to think about and look forward to. After his first Friendly Companion left after a year, he appropriately discussed feelings of loss with the Social Work Coordinator and staff, and readily accepted a new volunteer.

Youth volunteers have added a special component to the program, with veteran's noting "they brighten up the place." One youth volunteer responded to the interest of veterans by bringing in WWII magazines to discuss, and several others have assisted the resident in learning the computer and Internet. Another played piano for all veterans following his individual meetings with assigned patients. One veteran has viewed his meetings with youth volunteers as an opportunity to "help them out" by providing them with history, teaching them games, and making them feel comfortable during the visit. During an interview prior to his involvement with the Friendly Companion program, this patient had expressed a need to feel useful and it appears he enjoys the role this provides him. Residents have noted that the youth volunteers are very mature, and that is it "nice to see kids interested in what they are doing." For youths, the assignment is somewhat different in that all assigned residents are typically higher functioning and verbal. In some cases, youth volunteers have chosen to see patients in pairs, as this increases comfort level since this is a new experience for many who have chosen to volunteer.

Results of the Social Work Indicator do confirm that careful consideration regarding resident needs and volunteer abilities and personality are critical in determining an appropriate assignment, which will be mutually satisfying and result in retaining volunteers. From resident comments, it is clear that the matching of youth or adult volunteer is important in that some residents respond better to an older companion and some prefer a youth companion. One veteran also noted that he prefers volunteers who are not "overly sweet" as he perceived this as sympathy. As a result of this feedback, the Social Work Coordinator has provided additional training to volunteers regarding communication style. By observation, some male veterans also appear to interact best with male volunteers who are more direct and outgoing. In addition to gender considerations, personality seems to be an important factor in suitable matches.

Results from patient satisfaction surveys have also mentioned that time of day for the visit and length of the visit is important to patient satisfaction. Visits range anywhere from fifteen minutes for less responsive patients, to an hour or more for higher functioning and interactive patients. Time of day appears to depend on individual schedules, which considers appointments, unit activities, and times the patient wishes to spend resting. Social Work intervention is helpful in assisting residents in deciding what time of day they prefer to have the visits and for how long.

As termination of a Friendly Companion volunteer may stimulate abandonment issues, Social Work has provided intervention with the termination process in cases where the Friendly Companion must leave. The average length of service for adult Friendly Companion volunteers is about a year, with several approaching two years, and one who has been involved since inception of the program. Adult volunteers generally cite medical or family issues as primary reasons for leaving, and sometimes chose to leave after assigned patients have expired. Youths generally provide about three to four months of service, which corresponds to length of school assignment and summer breaks, with some staying on during the school year. Anticipated length of service commitment for volunteers is used in determining matches for residents to minimize abandonment issues, especially for youth volunteers. All volunteers are asked for ongoing feedback and complete an exit interview upon termination from the program, as volunteer satisfaction and retention remains an important area for Performance improvement.

FUTURE DIRECTIONS AND CONCLUSIONS

Several groups have expressed interest in being part of the Friendly Companion Program, including both seniors and youth. One of the current Friendly Companions is in the process of organizing a senior group at his local synagogue to become companions to give them something meaningful to do on a regular basis. A local school has also requested to bring a class of students to meet ongoing with patients. Patients were asked about this possibility, and all responded that they would welcome the opportunity to share stories and history with students. It is also hoped to expand the program to other onsite Nursing Home Care Units that may benefit from services, including the Palliative Care Unit.

In conclusion, the Friendly Companion program offers the opportunity for both patients and volunteers to form relationships that are satisfying and fulfilling, while improving overall clinical care and well being of institutionalized elders. It appears that the positive effects of Friendly Companion relationship generalize to overall increased social functioning. Residents appear to become more involved in other unit activities, and interact more with peers and staff. This program represents a multi-disciplinary effort to enhance patient care and maximize the quality of life of Nursing Home residents.

FRIENDLY COMPANION PROGRAM

Overview of Process

1. Voluntary Service refers potential volunteers to Friendly Companion Social Work Coordinator.
2. Social Work Coordinator screens volunteers and makes a decision regarding acceptance to program, or refers back to Voluntary Service with assessment/recommendations.

If accepted, Social Work Program Coordinator sets up an initial Screening, which includes:

a. Orientation/Refer to orientation checklist.
b. Tour and introductions to staff
c. Return to Voluntary Service to receive ID badge/youth jacket/parking stickers.
d. Follow up of Voluntary Service packets (post test), and PPD Screen.

3. On the first day, the Social Work Coordinator works very closely with the volunteer and first discusses the assignment and patients he/she will be working with. The assignments have been matched carefully according to patient needs and volunteer abilities. Social Work introduces the volunteer to the patients (who have agreed to

participate in an earlier information meeting with Social Work Coordinator). The volunteer meets with the Social Work Coordinator after each patient meeting on the first day to discuss questions, etc., Social Work Coordinator works very closely with the volunteer in the first few weeks and provides assistance and assignment changes as indicated.

4. Social Work Coordinator remains on site and available during Friendly Companion Visits, and provides ongoing supervision and education.

5. Social Work Coordinator continues to complete ongoing evaluations provided by Voluntary Service, which is a JCAHO requirement.

6. Social Work Coordinator uses a log to mark volunteer hours, which are then given to Voluntary Service.

7. Social Workers who have patients with assigned Friendly Companions note this program on the individual care plan and discuss in IDT meetings. During team Meetings, all patients are assessed for participation in FC program and referrals made.

8. Residents who participate are asked for their feedback every six months when Social Work Coordinator completes a Performance Indicator utilizing a Resident Satisfaction Survey.

REFERENCES

Gould, M.T. (1992). Nursing Home Elderly: Social-Environmental Factors. *Journal of Gerontological Nursing*, 18 (8) 13-20.

Greene,V.L., & Monahan, D.(1982). The Impact of Visitation on Patient Well-Being in Nursing Homes. *The Gerontologist*, 22(4) 418-423.

Gueldner, S.H. et al. (2001). Patterns of Telephone Use Among Nursing Home Residents. *Journal of Gerontological Nursing*, 27(5) 35-41.

Hicks, T.J. (2000) What is Your Life Like Now? Loneliness and Elderly Individuals Residing in Nursing Homes. *Journal of Gerontological Nursing*, 26 (8) 15-19.

Mitchell, J.M., and Kemp, B.J. (2000). Quality of Life in Assisted Living Homes: A Multidimensional Analysis. *Journal of Gerontology*: Psychological Sciences, 55B. 117-127.

Patterson, B.J. (1995). The Process of Social Support: Adjusting to Life in A Nursing Home. *Journal of Advanced Nursing*, 21, 682-689.

Port, C.L., & Baldini-Gruber et al. (2001). Resident Contact with Family and Friends Following Nursing Home Admission. *The Gerontologist*, 41, 589-596.

Windriver,W. (1993). Social Isolation: Unit Based Activities for Impaired Elders. *Journal of Gerontological Nursing*. 19 (3) 15-21.

Stories Told and Lessons Learned from African American Female Caregivers' Vignettes for Empowerment Practice

Letha A. Chadiha, PhD
Portia Adams, MSW
Odireleng Phorano, MSW
Seow Ling Ong, MSW
Lisa Byers, MSW

SUMMARY. In a group context, African American women told stories about their caregiving experiences. We audiotaped these stories and constructed vignettes that served as cases from the field. Lessons learned from vignettes about challenges and strengths in caregiving inform em-

---

Letha A. Chadiha is Associate Professor, University of Michigan-Ann Arbor, School of Social Work, Ann Arbor. She received funding from the John A. Hartford Geriatric Social Work Faculty Scholars' Program for this manuscript. Portia Adams is a doctoral candidate at George Warren Brown School of Social Work, Washington University-St. Louis. Odireleng Phorano is Social Work Faculty of social sciences at the University of Botswana-Gaborone. Seow Ling Ong is Research Associate at Education, Training and Research Associates, San Francisco, CA. Lisa Byers is a doctoral student at George Warren Brown School of Social Work, Washington University-St. Louis.

David Biegel, National Mentor, Hartford Geriatric Social Work Faculty Scholars' Program, and Jane Rafferty gave helpful comments. Emmanuel Akuamoah, Alice Ansah-Koi, Swapna Kommidi, and Pramod Pandey provided technical assistance.

[Haworth co-indexing entry note]: "Stories Told and Lessons Learned from African American Female Caregivers' Vignettes for Empowerment Practice." Chadiha, Letha A., et al. Co-published simultaneously in *Journal of Gerontological Social Work* (The Haworth Social Work Practice Press, an imprint of The Haworth Press, Inc.) Vol. 40, No. 1/2, 2002, pp. 135-144; and: *Older People and Their Caregivers Across the Spectrum of Care* (ed: Judith L. Howe) The Haworth Social Work Practice Press, an imprint of The Haworth Press, Inc., 2003, pp. 135-144. Single or multiple copies of this article are available for a fee from The Haworth Document Delivery Service [1-800-HAWORTH, 9:00 a.m. - 5:00 p.m. (EST). E-mail address: docdelivery@haworthpress.com].

http://www.haworthpress.com/store/product.asp?sku=J083
10.1300/J083v40n01_09

powerment group practice with African American women caregivers of African American elders. *[Article copies available for a fee from The Haworth Document Delivery Service: 1-800-HAWORTH. E-mail address: <docdelivery@haworthpress.com> Website: <http://www.HaworthPress.com> © 2002 by The Haworth Press, Inc. All rights reserved.]*

KEYWORDS. African American, caregivers, elders, empowerment, group practice, informal care, narratives, storytelling, strengths, vignettes

INTRODUCTION AND BACKGROUND

Informal caregiving is unpaid help with basic personal needs, chores, errands, and transportation provided by relatives and non-relatives to older adults (Johnson & Lo Sasso, 2001), typically persons 65 years old or more residing in the community (Feder, Komisar, & Niefeld, 2000). African American women, mainly daughters, provide the bulk of informal care to community-dwelling older African American adults (National Alliance for Caregiving & American Association of Retired Persons, 1997). While these women demonstrate strengths through strong coping with challenging caregiving tasks and report caregiving as rewarding (Connell & Gibson, 1997; Dilworth-Anderson, Williams, & Gibson, 2002; Janevic & Connell, 2001; Picot, 1995; Picot, Debanne, Namazi, & Wykle, 1997), they rely less on problem-solving coping and more on emotion-focused coping, a type of coping associated with mental health costs in caregiving (Knight, Silverstein, McCallum, & Fox, 2000). Literature further suggests that African American women caregivers may experience both physical health (Grason, Minkovitz, Misra, & Strobino, 2001) and economic costs in caregiving (Arno, Levine, & Memmott, 1999; Johnson & Lo Sasso, 2001). Taking these costs in caregiving into consideration, we developed an empowerment group intervention in a larger study for African American women caregivers of African American elders (Chadiha, 1999).

Empowerment, according to Gutierrez (1994), is the "process of increasing personal, interpersonal, or political power so that individuals, families, and communities can take action to improve their situations" (p. 202). In an effort to empower themselves, people may take individual action and join with others in a group in order to improve challenging life situations (Lee, 2001). Empowerment literature on women, people of color (Cox & Parsons, 1996; Gutierrez, 1990; Lee, 2001; Lewis, 1999) and older adults (Cox, 1989) provides a rationale for an empowerment approach to practice with African American women caregivers. This literature offers a lens for understanding how African American women may seek to take charge of their lives in challenging and undesirable caregiving situations.

In this paper, we examined three vignettes as cases from the field in order to learn about the process of empowerment for African American women caregivers in a group context. Specifically, we examined these vignettes for both strengths and challenges in caregiving. Clark (2002) has noted "case studies are used extensively in gerontological and geriatric education and practice, especially to present clinically relevant examples and to illustrate abstract concepts, principles, and theories in the study of aging" (p. 297). In a similar vein, vignettes as field cases serve not only to inform gerontological social work practice but also to illustrate principles of empowerment practice with African American women caregivers.

METHODS: RECRUITMENT, SAMPLE, DATA GATHERING AND ANALYSIS

Vignettes, in the current study, were based on data collected for a larger study that aimed to test the applicability and feasibility of an empowerment intervention with African American women caregivers of African American elders (Chadiha, 1999). Women were eligible for participation in this larger study if they identified as African American, were 18 years old and older, had not participated in a support group, and provided unpaid care to an African American elder (60 years old or more) without an Alzheimer's diagnosis. We recruited caregivers by announcing the study in an African American newspaper, the newsletter of an African American church, on a local television station and by disseminating flyers to local community agencies serving older African American adults. Participants also referred caregivers. Caregivers received $50 for full participation in the larger study.

A majority of the 23 African American female caregivers in the larger study were unmarried (96%) daughters (74%) of the care recipient. Just less than half of the caregivers were working (45%) outside the home and living with the elderly person (48%). Slightly more than half had spent one to five years caring for the elderly person (56%). Caregivers had an average age of 46 years (SD = 14.70) and average educational level of 13 years (SD = 2.19).

We relied on the narrative or storytelling approach to collect caregivers' stories in a group context. Narrative literature indicates that when people tell stories they are constructing meaning–making sense out of challenging life experiences, raising awareness of those experiences, reevaluating challenging life experiences as a motive for change, and identifying personal strengths in adverse circumstances (Borden, 1992; Mishler, 1986). Use of the storytelling approach in a group was guided by Rappaport's (1995) conceptualization of the "community narrative," a shared story among a group of people. It was also guided by the notion that a group approach to storytelling embraced elements of empowerment such as collaboration, inclusiveness, and mutual support (Rappaport, 1995). In order to construct vignettes, we listened to the audiotaped stories of caregivers collected in two-hour group meetings during the first three weeks of a seven-week empowerment group program. An African American female doctoral social work student, with a master of social work degree and group work experience, facilitated the group meetings. In a general sense, we employed an inductive approach to construct vignettes by using the facts in the stories of caregivers (Tutty, Rothery, & Grinnell, 1996). From a practical standpoint, we chose vignettes that illustrate both strengths and challenges in caregivers' stories. The concept of strengths refers to the ability of people to use both psychological coping and tangible resources in order to transform adverse life situations into nurturing situations, whereas the concept of challenges refers to life situations that threaten the ability of people to actualize and affirm their lives (Lee, 2001).

CASES FROM THE FIELD

Vignette #1

Ms. Porter is an attractive, divorced, middle-aged African American woman who retired from her job of twenty years and lives alone. She has adult children and grandchildren who live out of state. She cares for her mother, Mrs. Davis, who is the much beloved matriarch of the Davis and Porter families. She is 91 years old, in good health, a stylish dresser, and a regular church attendee. She lives on a pension and is ineligible for Medicaid services.

Ms. Porter explained to the group that she visits her mother daily. Every morning she gets up, drives to her mother's home, and makes her breakfast and dinner. She helps with groceries, laundry, banking, medications, and medical appointments. Ms. Porter also helps purchase her mother's medications, which is a financial challenge she bears. Ms. Porter believes that family should care for family and in comparison to some caregivers–her burden is not that heavy. Yet she misses time for her own life. It seems that her mother wants her to be at her beckon call.

In the group, she realized that sometimes she feels resentful and guilty because she thinks she shouldn't get aggravated, as she states "This is my mother." Ms. Porter had not noticed how resentful she felt about caring for her mother until she talked about it in the group. The group members empathized with Ms. Porter's loss of autonomy, acknowledged her feelings, her contributions, the financial burden, and her need for time away from caring for her mother. During her time in the group, Ms. Porter began to negotiate with her mother for more time of her own and to encourage her brother to assist in her care. Ms. Porter also suggested to the group that the government must assist elders without comprehensive health benefits, especially for the costs of equipment and medications.

Vignette #2

Ms. Ware is an energetic, older African American woman. She is the eldest daughter, a widow with several adult children and grandchildren. Ms. Ware moved into her mother's home after her father died and her mother, Mrs. Roberts, started to have health problems. Ms. Ware and her mother enjoy each other's company and frequently play board games together. Mrs. Roberts used to be very independent, and a sharp dresser. In the past she and her daughter would often travel together. Ms. Ware explained, "We would fuss and laugh with each other. I tell her off and she tells me off. She has a mind of her own, and you don't want to be disrespectful. You want to do the right thing." Ms. Ware's family helps care for her mother: "I have the highest confidence in my brothers and they have helped a lot. But she really likes me (Mrs. Roberts) so she is mostly with me."

As Ms. Ware recounts her caregiving experience the other members of the group note that Ms. Ware has been a caregiver most of her life and that she does the job well. Ms. Ware cared for a child with a chronic mental illness, she cared for her husband for years before he died, and now she is taking care of her mother. It is clear that Ms. Ware enjoys caring for her mother but she has some concerns. Ms. Ware has her own physical health issues, and she is sometimes confused by her mother's complicated medical program. Ms. Ware is also concerned about preserving their mother-daughter relationship, and respecting her mother's authority and independence.

Ms. Ware garnered respect within the group and helped members recognize that older adults need autonomy. She reminded members how African American families in her community cared for elders in the past. She spoke of the cultural ties that the group members shared. At the same time she was aware that the family support she received was not a common experience for other members of the group. She engaged members in discussions about how things have changed in their families and helped members to brainstorm solutions to problems in caregiving. She was also connected to an elderly advocacy group to assist with clarifying and implementing her mother's medical program.

Vignette #3

Ms. Bond is a plump and pleasant middle-aged African American woman, divorced, and lives with her mother and a teenage daughter. Ms. Bond works full-time at a social service agency. An only child, Ms. Bond had a difficult relationship with her mother even prior to her mother's disability. Ms. Bond has been taking care of her mother for seven years. She explained to the group that she often feels motivated by guilt to care for her mother. When her mother asks for something, Ms. Bond believes that she should drop everything to get her mother what she wants. She says: "Momma is not as she used to be. Now she is not able to do for herself." And sometimes Ms. Bond worries: What if her mother were to die today? So Ms. Bond states that if there is any thing her mother wants, she gets it.

Yet it seems that her mother has a lot of needs and that her work never ends. Ms. Bond cried, "I'm tired. I'm ready to move. I am not content. I am tired. My child is not doing well at school and I fussed with her, I went on and on. All that fussing was not necessary, my frustration was toward my mother and I was taking it out on my child." Ms. Bond told the group that once she went to visit some nursing homes and her aunt accused her of wanting to "throw my mother away."

This information about Ms. Bond's experience started a lively group discussion about whether African American people place their old persons in nursing homes. All agreed that if an elder was very disabled and they could not provide proper care, a nursing home would be a final resort. The group empathized with her dilemma, the guilt and the exhaustion of bringing up a teenager and caring for her mother at the same time. Ms. Bond is very religious. She told the group that when she goes to church she feels relief and comfort. "I feel like a whole burden is lifted off of me. Because I believe that once you put it in His hands, you can't worry about it anymore." The group echoed this belief and members spoke of how God had gotten them through the hard times. Ms. Bond also confided that the group was "her time for herself."

DISCUSSION

Viewed through the lens of an empowerment approach to practice, empowerment is a process in which people engage to improve their lives by changing challenging life situations into positive change (Gutierrez, 1994; Lee, 2001). Empowerment practice emphasizes letting vulnerable clients tell their stories, educating them to define their problems, promoting their collaborative actions to solve common problems, and building on their existing strengths (Cox & Parsons, 1996; Gutierrez, 1990; Lee, 2001). People are placed in an ideal position to empower themselves through taking individual actions and working collaboratively with others to solve problems. Social workers facilitate the empowerment process of clients by letting them identify problems, providing a supportive group context for clients to work with other people to solve problems, and drawing upon the strengths of clients as a resource for facilitating positive change in their lives (Gutierrez, 1990; Lee, 2001).

Vignettes as field cases yield several lessons for empowerment social work practice with African American women caregivers of older adult family members. First, storytelling allows these women to speak in their own voices about caregiving experiences. Specifically, storytelling offers them opportunity to identify, define, and focus on problems of interest to them rather than focus on problems of interest to the group facilitator. Problems of caregiving are identified and defined through reports of Ms. Porter's lack of time for her own life, Ms. Ware's care responsibility for multiple family members, and the prodigious care needs of Ms. Bond's mother. Second, because scholars regard the small group as an ideal modality for empowerment practice (Gutierrez, 1990; Lee, 2001) a group context offers opportunity for African American women to work collaboratively with other caregivers to identify solutions to problems. Group members, for example, help validate concerns of Ms. Porter about feeling resentful for the amount of time she has to spend caring for her mother and wanting to have more time for her self-care. Third, we learn through the interactions of African American women with other group members that caregivers are motivated to advocate not only for change within the caregiving situation but also to advocate for change within the service delivery system. Ms. Porter, for example, negotiates with her mother for time out from caregiving and encourages her sibling to assist with their mother's care. Ms. Ware participates in an advocacy group in order to facilitate discussions with her mother's medical provider and help clarify as well as simplify her mother's complicated medical program. Fourth, although literature suggests that African American caregivers as a group may underuse formal services such as nursing home care (Yeo, 1993), the women explore the topic of African Americans and nursing home placement for older adults. While caregivers agree that placing a family member in a nursing home would be a final resort for them personally, the fact that the women are spontaneously addressing this topic would suggest that they are aware of the potential need for nursing home placement as a care option for loved ones. Last, concomitantly with the women's reports of challenges in caregiving are strengths such as strong religious coping (Ms. Bond's statement of feeling relief and comfort in church) and mastery of multiple caregiving roles (Ms. Ware's accounts of caring for a child with a chronic mental illness and caring for her husband who is now deceased) that serve as a resource to African American women caregivers.

In conclusion, vignettes based on stories that African American women caregivers told in a group context provide a medium for understanding challenges and strengths in caregiving to an older adult family member. While it is unrealistic to think African American women are empowered after meeting three times in a group, the mutual support that these women gain from being with similar others in a group context becomes an invaluable resource for transforming challenging caregiving into positive change.

There may be limitations to using a group narrative or storytelling approach with caregivers. This approach may generate fear for some participants, risk exposing what some participants may regard as personal failures in caring for loved ones, and risk one person's story becoming dominant over another person's story. Empowerment theory suggests, however, that a group context will enhance collaboration, trust, and sharing of power among African American women caregivers (Gutierrez & Lewis, 1999). Being in a group with similar others may facilitate risk-taking in a way that the dyadic therapeutic format cannot simulate for these women caregivers.

Vignettes are limited inasmuch as they are constructed accounts of reality and may deviate from the original accounts of storytellers (Clark, 2002). Still, vignettes as field cases are recognized as a useful teaching and practice tool for gerontological social workers. They provide gerontological social workers with lenses for understanding challenges, strengths, and empowerment principles such as collaboration and mutual support for African American women caregivers. The process of empowerment for African American women caregivers may be more a journey than a destination. Most important, that journey may have begun when the women in this study chose to join a group and talk about their experiences with women of similar race and caregiving experience.

REFERENCES

Arno, P. S., Levine, C., & Memmott, M. M. (1999). The economic value of informal caregiving. *Health Affairs, 18*, 182-188.

Borden, W. (1992). Narrative perspective in psychosocial interventions following adverse life events. *Social Work, 37*, 135-141.

Chadiha, L. A. (1999). Beyond coping: An empowerment intervention for African American women caregivers of dependent elders. Unpublished manuscript.

Clark, P. G. (2002). Values and voices in teaching gerontology and geriatrics: Case studies as stories. *The Gerontologist, 42*, 297-303.

Connell, C. M., & Gibson, G. D. (1997). Racial, ethnic, and cultural differences in dementia caregiving: Review and analysis. *The Gerontologist, 37*, 355-364.

Cox, E. O. (1989). Empowerment of the low income elderly through group work. *Social Work with Groups, 11*, 111-125.

Cox, E. O., & Parsons, R. J. (1996). Empowerment oriented social work practice: Impact on late life relationships with women. *Journal of Women and Aging, 8*, 129-143.

Dilworth-Anderson, P., Williams, W.S., & Gibson, B. E. (2002). Issues of race, ethnicity, and culture in caregiving research: A 20-year review (1980-2000). *The Gerontologist, 42*, 237-272.

Feder, J., Komisar, H.L., & Niefeld, M. (2000). Long term care in the United States: An overview. *Health Affairs, 19*, 40-56.

Grason, H., Minkovitz, C., Misra, D., & Strobino, D. (2001). Impact of social and economic factors on women's health. In D. Misra (Ed.), *The women's health data book: A profile of women's health in the United States* (pp. 2-13). Washington, DC: Jacobs Institute of Women's Health & The Henry J. Kaiser Family Foundation. Third Edition.

Gutierrez, L. (1990). Working with women of color: An empowerment perspective. *Social Work, 35*, 149-154.

Gutierrez, L. (1994). Beyond coping: An empowerment perspective on stressful life events. *Journal of Sociology and Social Welfare, 21*, 201-219.

Gutierrez, L., & Lewis, E.A. (1999). *Empowering women of color.* New York: Columbia University Press.

Janevic, M. R., & Connell, C. M. (2001). Racial, ethnic, and cultural differences in the dementia caregiving experience: Recent findings. *The Gerontologist, 41,* 334-347.

Johnson, R.W., & Lo Sasso, A. T. (2001). The employment and time costs of caring for elderly parents. *Poverty Research News, 5,* 5-7.

Knight, B. G., Silverstein, M., McCallum, T. J., & Fox, L. S. (2000). A psychological stress and coping model for mental health among African American caregivers in Southern California. *Journal of Gerontology: Psychological Sciences, 55B,* 142-150.

Lewis, E. (1999). Staying on the path: Lessons about health and resistance from women of the African diaspora in the United States. In L.M. Gutierrez and E. Lewis (Eds.), *Empowering women of color* (pp. 150-166). New York: Columbia Press.

Lee, J.A. (2001). *The empowerment approach to social work practice. Building the beloved community.* New York: Columbia University Press. Second edition.

Maxwell, J. A. (1992). Understanding and validity in qualitative research. *Harvard Educational Review, 62,* 279-300.

Mishler, E. (1986). *Research interviewing: Context and narrative.* Cambridge, MA: Harvard University Press.

National Alliance for Caregiving and American Association of Retired Persons. (1997). *Family caregiving in the U.S.: Findings from a national survey.* Bethesda, MD: National Alliance for Caregiving & American Association of Retired Persons.

Picot, S. J. (1995). Rewards, costs, and coping of African-American caregivers. *Nursing Research, 44,* 147-152.

Picot, S. J., Debanne, S. M., Namazi, K. H., & Wykle, M. L. (1997). Religiosity and perceived rewards of Black and White caregivers. *The Gerontologist, 37,* 89-101.

Rappaport, J. (1995). Empowerment meets narrative: Listening to stories and creating settings. *American Journal of Community Psychology, 23,* 795-807.

Tutty, L.M., Rothery, M., & Grinnell, R. M. (1996). *Qualitative research for social workers.* Boston: Allyn and Bacon.

Yeo, G.W. (1993). Ethnicity and nursing homes: Factors affecting use and successful components for culturally sensitive care. In C.M. Barresi & D.E. Stull (Eds.), *Ethnic elderly and long-term care* (pp. 161-177). New York: Springer Publishing.

Index

AARP/Travelers Foundation caregiver study, 64-65
Abuse. *See* Elder abuse
Abuser impairment, 85
Activities of Daily Living. *See* ADLs; IADLs
Activities of Daily Living Index, 18
ADLs
 assessment, 47-48
 in HIV/AIDS, 50-51,54-56
 On Lok (PACE) assessment model, 18
 long-distance caregiver survey, 71
African-American female caregivers, 135-144. *See also* Empowerment practice
Age. *See* Demographics
Ageism, 46,57
AIDS. *See* HIV/AIDS
(University of) Alabama, 101-121. *See also* Life Course Model of Parent Care
Alzheimer's Association, 29
Alzheimer's disease, 51,56
 family caregivers and, 28-29,31-32
American Association of Retired Persons (AARP), 64,65. *See also* NAC/AARP national survey
Antiretroviral therapy, age ratios, 57
Assessment, 1-14
 abuse, 11-12
 ADLs/IADLs, 47-48
 biopsychosocial context, 5-6
 caregiver health and burden, 50
 cognitive, 9-10,48
 culturally sensitive, 7-8
 current healthcare context, 3-6
 early research on, 2-3
 emotional status, 48

end-of-life issues, 12
follow-up, 29
functional, 9
geriatric, 47-50
grief and loss, 11
in HIV/AIDS, 41-62,50-58
hospital-related problems, 11
On Lok (PACE) model, 17-19
major factors, 9-12
medications, 49
Parent Care Readiness, 114
psychological, 9
sexuality, 49
social support, 10-11,48
spirituality, 49
standardized instruments, 6-7,18

Best practice, On Lok (PACE) model, 15-22
(University of) Botswana-Gabarone, 135-144. *See also* Empowerment practice
Brief Multidimensional Measure of Religiousness and Spirituality, 49
Brigham Young University, 101-121. *See also* Life Course Model of Parent Care

CAPP. *See* Caregivers and Professionals Partnership (CAPP)
Caregiver burden, 50,66-67,74
 distance-related difficulty, 74-76
 elder abuse and, 84
 employment-related, 71-74
 in HIV/AIDS, 54,57

Race/ethnicity. *See* Demographics
Religion and spirituality, 49

Safety outcomes, in elder abuse, 94-98
Secondary caregivers, 65
Self-identification, 34-35,36
Sexuality assessment, 49,52
  in HIV/AIDS, 56-57
Sexuality-related language, 57
Short Portable Mental Status
    Questionnaire, 18
Social support
    assessment, 48
  in HIV/AIDS, 52,56
  long-distance caregivers, 77
Solano County (California) Health and
    Social Services, 41-62. *See
    also* HIV/AIDS
Spirituality assessment, 49,52
STEPS (Services to Empower
    Seniors), 86. *See also* Elder
    abuse
Stress, caregiver. *See* Caregiver burden
Survivor guilt, 46

Tinetti Balance and Gait Scale, 18
Turning points, in life course, 106

University of Alabama, 101-121. *See
    also* Life Course Model of
    Parent Care
University of Botswana-Gabarone,
    135-144
University of Michigan-Ann Arbor,
    135-144. *See also*
    Empowerment practice

University of Washington (Tacoma),
    41-62. *See also* HIV/AIDS
US Army/US Air Force War College,
    101-121. *See also* Life
    Course Model of Parent Care

VAMC Northport Nursing Home
    Friendly Companion
    Program, 123-135. *See also*
    Friendly Companion
    Program
Venereal disease, as term, 57
Vignettes, as study method, 135-144
Virginia Commonwealth University,
    63-81. *See also*
    Long-distance caregivers
Volunteers. *See* Friendly Companion
    Program

Walk the Walk, Inc., 83-100. *See also*
    Elder abuse
(University of) Washington (Tacoma),
    41-62. *See also* HIV/AIDS
Washington University-St. Louis,
    135-144. *See also*
    Empowerment practice
Well Spouse Foundation, 29
Women. *See also* Gender differences
    African-American informal
    caregivers, 135-144 (*See also*
    Empowerment practice)
    employed as caregivers, 101-121
    (*See also* Life Course Model
    of Parent Care)

Youth volunteers, 130. *See also*
    Friendly Companion
    Program